ABC OF PRETERM BIRTH

ABC OF PRETERM BIRTH

Edited by

WILLIAM McGUIRE

*Senior lecturer in neonatal medicine, Tayside Institute of Child Health,
Ninewells Hospital and Medical School, Dundee*

and

PETER W FOWLIE

Consultant paediatrician, Perth Royal Infirmary, and Ninewells Hospital and Medical School, Dundee

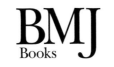

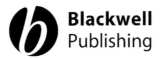

© 2005 by Blackwell Publishing Ltd
BMJ Books is an imprint of the BMJ Publishing Group Limited, used under licence

Blackwell Publishing, Inc., 350 Main Street, Malden, Massachusetts 02148-5020, USA
Blackwell Publishing Ltd, 9600 Garsington Road, Oxford OX4 2DQ, UK
Blackwell Publishing Asia Pty Ltd, 550 Swanston Street, Carlton, Victoria 3053, Australia

First published 2005

Library of Congress Cataloging-in-Publication Data
ABC of preterm birth/edited by William McGuire, Peter W. Fowlie.
   p. ; cm.
 Includes bibliographical references and index.
 ISBN-13: 978-0-7279-1763-8
 ISBN-10: 0-7279-1763-3
 1. Infants, Premature—Medical care. 2. Infants, Premature—Care. 3. Postnatal care. 4. Labor,
Premature.
 [DNLM: 1. Perinatal Care—methods. 2. Premature Birth. 3. Infant, Newborn, Diseases—therapy.
4. Infant, Premature.] I. McGuire, William, 1963– II. Fowlie, Peter W.

RJ250.A23 2005
618.92′01—dc22

200500069

ISBN-13: 978 0 7279 1763 8
ISBN-10: 0 7279 1763 3

A catalogue record for this title is available from the British Library

The cover shows a premature (neonatal) infant delivered during the seventh month of pregnancy.
With permission from Petit Format/Science Photo Library

Set by BMJ Electronic Production
Printed and bound in Spain by GraphyCems, Navarra

Commissioning Editor: Eleanor Lines
Development Editors: Sally Carter/Nick Morgan
Production Controller: Debbie Wyer

For further information on Blackwell Publishing, visit our website:
http://www.blackwellpublishing.com

The publisher's policy is to use permanent paper from mills that operate a sustainable forestry policy, and
which has been manufactured from pulp processed using acid-free and elementary chlorine-free practices.
Furthermore, the publisher ensures that the text paper and cover board used have met acceptable
environmental accreditation standards.

Contents

Contributors

Philip Booth
Consultant paediatrician, Aberdeen Maternity Hospital, Aberdeen

Peter Brocklehurst
Director of the National Perinatal Epidemiology Unit, Institute of Health Sciences, Oxford

Linda Clerihew
Specialist registrar, neonatal intensive care unit, Ninewells Hospital and Medical School, Dundee

Michael Colvin
Consultant paediatrician, Stirling Royal Infirmary, Stirling

Peter W Fowlie
Consultant paediatrician, Perth Royal Infirmary and Ninewells Hospital and Medical School, Dundee

Jenny Fraser
Specialist registrar, neonatal intensive care unit, Ninewells Hospital and Medical School, Dundee

Ginny Henderson
Research nurse, school of nursing and midwifery, University of Dundee

Peter McEwan
Specialist registrar, neonatal intensive care unit, Ninewells Hospital and Medical School, Dundee

William McGuire
Senior lecturer in neonatal medicine, Tayside Institute of Child Health, Ninewells Hospital and Medical School, Dundee

Hazel McHaffie
Deputy director of research, Institute of Medical Ethics, Loanhead, Midlothian

Deirdre J Murphy
Professor of obstetrics and gynaecology, Maternal and Child Health Sciences, Ninewells Hospital and Medical School, Dundee

Gareth Parry
Senior research fellow, Medical Care Research Unit, School of Health and Related Research, University of Sheffield

Charles H Skeoch
Consultant paediatrician, Princess Royal Maternity Hospital, Glasgow

Janet Tucker
Senior researcher at the Dugald Baird Centre, department of obstetrics and gynaecology, University of Aberdeen

Moira Walls
Neonatal nurse, neonatal intensive care unit, Ninewells Hospital and Medical School, Dundee

Foreword

The final quarter of the last century saw enormous developments in the care of sick newborn babies, particularly those born before their due date. Although survival and good outcome is now universally expected for babies born a few weeks early, those born before 32 weeks' gestation are often less fortunate and may either die or survive with long term neurological and developmental problems.

Perinatal medicine, spanning the care of mothers at risk of preterm delivery, intrapartum care, and the full range of neonatal medicine, is now firmly established as an integrated discipline of medicine. Nevertheless, the team is large and each member may have a specialised role. Ensuring that a mother receives timely advice and care, and that decisions are communicated effectively, is essential. A fine balance has to be struck between the risks and benefits, and so the planning and timing of preterm delivery is often crucial.

After a shaky start that led to some disasters in management, care before and after preterm delivery has been subjected to a wide range of well conducted large randomised controlled trials. Evidence continues to accumulate through multicentre studies, and this will refine our understanding of the benefits and hazards of new treatments.

In the *ABC of Preterm Birth*, Bill McGuire, Peter Fowlie, and their colleagues have produced a comprehensive guide to all the main issues of preterm births. This book will be essential to all who play a part in the perinatal team. As more preterm babies survive to discharge, the carers in the community, general practitioners, and health visitors, as well as other paediatricians and a wide range of specialists to whom preterm babies may later be referred, will find the book to be an invaluable source of facts and sensible information.

Andrew R Wilkinson
Professor of Paediatrics
University of Oxford
John Radcliffe Hospital
Oxford

1 Epidemiology of preterm birth

Janet Tucker, William McGuire

Preterm birth is a major challenge in perinatal health care. Most perinatal deaths occur in preterm infants, and preterm birth is an important risk factor for neurological impairment, including cerebral palsy. Preterm birth not only affects infants and their families—providing care for preterm infants, who may spend several months in hospital, has increasing cost implications for health services.

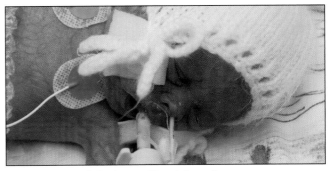

Extremely preterm infant born at 26 weeks' gestation

Definitions

Preterm birth is the delivery of a baby before 37 completed weeks' gestation. Most mortality and morbidity affects "very preterm" infants (those born before 32 weeks' gestation), and especially "extremely preterm" infants (those born before 28 weeks of gestation).

Over the past 20-30 years advances in perinatal care have improved outcomes for infants born after short gestations. The number of weeks of completed gestation that defines whether a birth is preterm rather than a fetal loss has become smaller. In 1992 the boundary that required registration as a preterm live birth in the United Kingdom was lowered from 28 completed weeks' gestation to 24 weeks' gestation. This boundary varies internationally, however, from about 20 to 24 weeks. Some classification of fetal loss, still birth, and early neonatal death for these very short gestations may be unreliable.

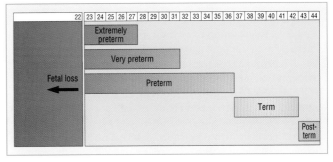

Definitions of preterm live births by completed weeks of gestation

Gestational age versus birth weight

Even in developed countries, there is often uncertainty and incomplete recording of estimates of gestation. In most of the United Kingdom data on birth weight data but not on gestational age are collected routinely.

Although some concordance exists between the categories of birth weight and gestational age, they are not interchangeable. The categories for birth weight are:
- Low birth weight (< 2500 g)
- Very low birth weight (< 1500 g)
- Extremely low birth weight (< 1000 g)

Only around two thirds of low birth weight infants are preterm. Term infants may be of low birth weight because they are "small for gestational age" or "light for date" infants. These infants are usually defined as below the 10th centile of the index population's distribution of birth weights by gestation—that is, in the lowest 10 per cent of birth weights.

Preterm infants may also be small for gestational age. They may have neonatal problems additional to those related to shortened gestation, particularly if they are small because of intrauterine growth restriction.

Perinatal problems related to intrauterine growth restriction include:
- Perinatal stress
- Fetal distress
- Meconium aspiration syndrome
- Hypoglycaemia
- Polycythaemia or hyperviscosity
- Hypothermia.

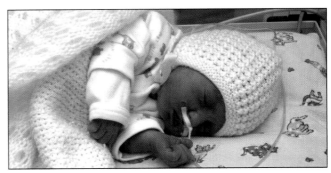

Preterm infant born at 35 weeks' gestation

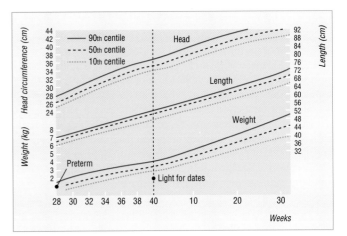

Chart for plotting progress of newborn infants' weight, head circumference, and length (with two examples)

1

Incidence

Over the past 20-30 years the incidence of preterm birth in most developed countries has been about 5-7% of live births. The incidence in the United States is higher, at about 12%. Some evidence shows that this incidence has increased slightly in the past few years, but the rate of birth before 32 weeks' gestation is almost unchanged, at 1-2%.

Several factors have contributed to the overall rise in the incidence of preterm birth. These factors include increasing rates of multiple births, greater use of assisted reproduction techniques, and more obstetric intervention.

Part of the apparent rise in the incidence of preterm birth, however, may reflect changes in clinical practice. Increasingly, ultrasonography rather than the last menstrual period date is used to estimate gestational age. The rise in incidence may also be caused by inconsistent classification of fetal loss, still birth, and early neonatal death. In some countries, infants who are born after very short gestations (less than 24 weeks) are more likely to be categorised as live births.

With the limited provision of antenatal or perinatal care in developing countries, there are difficulties with population based data. Registration of births is incomplete and information is lacking on gestational age, especially outside hospital settings. Data that are collected tend to give only estimates of perinatal outcomes that are specific to birth weight. These data show that the incidence of low birth weight is much higher in developing countries than in developed countries with good care services.

In developing counties, low birth weight is probably caused by intrauterine growth restriction. Maternal undernutrition and chronic infection in pregnancy are the main factors that cause intrauterine growth restriction. Although the technical advances in the care of preterm infants have improved outcomes in developed countries with well resourced care services, they have not influenced neonatal morbidity and mortality in countries that lack basic midwifery and obstetric care. In these developing countries, the priorities are to reduce infection associated with delivery, identify and manage pregnancies of women who are at risk, and provide basic neonatal resuscitation.

Causes of preterm birth

Spontaneous preterm labour and rupture of membranes
Most preterm births follow spontaneous, unexplained preterm labour, or spontaneous preterm prelabour rupture of the amniotic membranes. The most important factors that contribute to spontaneous preterm delivery are a history of preterm birth and poor socioeconomic background of the mother.

Interaction of the many factors that contribute to the association of preterm birth with socioeconomic status is complex. Mothers who smoke cigarettes are twice as likely as non-smoking mothers to deliver before 32 weeks of gestation, although this effect does not explain all the risk associated with social disadvantage.

Evidence from meta-analysis of randomised controlled trials shows that antenatal smoking cessation programmes can lower the incidence of preterm birth. Women from poorer socioeconomic backgrounds, however, are least likely to stop smoking in pregnancy although they are most at risk of preterm delivery.

No studies have shown that other interventions, such as better antenatal care, dietary advice, or increased social support during pregnancy, improve perinatal outcomes or reduce the social inequalities in the incidence of preterm delivery.

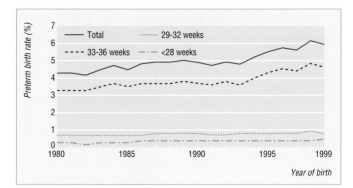

Rates of preterm birth, by gestational age, in singleton live births in New Zealand, 1980-99

Percentage of preterm births in United States*

| | Gestational age | |
Year	<37 weeks	<32 weeks
1981	9.4	1.81
1990	10.6	1.92
2000	11.6	1.93

*Adapted from MacDorman MF et al. *Pediatrics* 2002;110: 1037-52

Risk factors for babies with low birth weight in developing countries

- Infection, especially malaria
- Poor maternal nutrition
- Maternal anaemia
- Low maternal body mass index before pregnancy
- Short interval between pregnancies

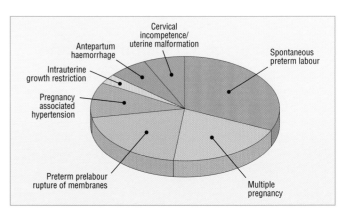

Causes of preterm birth

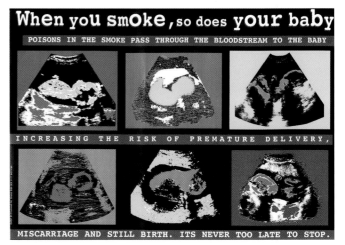

Smoking cessation programmes can lower the incidence of preterm birth

The rate of preterm birth varies between ethnic groups. In the United Kingdom, and even more markedly in the United States, the incidence of preterm birth in black women is higher than that in white women of similar age. The reason for this variation is unclear because differences remain after taking into account socioeconomic risk factors.

Multiple pregnancy and assisted reproduction

Multifetal pregnancy increases the risk of preterm delivery. About one quarter of preterm births occur in multiple pregnancies. Half of all twins and most triplets are born preterm. Multiple pregnancy is more likely than singleton pregnancy to be associated with spontaneous preterm labour and with preterm obstetric interventions, such as induction of labour or delivery by caesarean section.

The incidence of multiple pregnancies in developed countries has increased over the past 20-30 years. This rise is mainly because of the increased use of assisted reproduction techniques, such as drugs that induce ovulation and in vitro fertilisation. For example, the birth rate of twins in the United States has increased by 55% since 1980. The rate of higher order multiple births increased fourfold between 1980 and 1998, although this rate has decreased slightly over the past five years. In some countries two embryos only are allowed to be placed in the uterus after in vitro fertilisation to limit the incidence of higher order pregnancy.

Singleton pregnancies that follow assisted reproduction are at a considerable increased risk of preterm delivery, probably because of factors such as cervical trauma, the higher incidence of uterine problems, and possibly because of the increased risk of infection.

Maternal and fetal complications

About 15% to 25% of preterm infants are delivered because of maternal or fetal complications of pregnancy. The principal causes are hypertensive disorders of pregnancy and severe intrauterine growth restriction, which is often associated with hypertensive disorders. The decision to deliver these infants is informed by balancing the risks of preterm birth for the infant against the consequence of continued pregnancy for the mother and fetus. Over the past two decades improved antenatal and perinatal care has increased the rate of iatrogenic preterm delivery. During that time the incidence of still birth in the third trimester has fallen.

Outcomes after preterm birth

Broadly, outcomes improve with increasing gestational age, although for any given length of gestation survival varies with birth weight. Other factors, including ethnicity and gender also influence survival and the risk of neurological impairment.

The outcomes for preterm infants born at or after 32 weeks of gestation are similar to those for term infants. Most serious problems associated with preterm birth occur in the 1% to 2% of infants who are born before 32 completed weeks' gestation, and particularly the 0.4% of infants born before 28 weeks' gestation. Modern perinatal care and specific interventions, such as prophylactic antenatal steroids and exogenous surfactants, have contributed to some improved outcomes for very preterm infants. The overall prognosis remains poor, however, particularly for infants who are born before 26 weeks' gestation.

The outcome for preterm infants of multiple pregnancies can be better than that of singleton pregnancies of the same gestation. In term infants the situation is reversed. The

---

Preterm births by ethnic group in United States 2000*

- Black—17.3%
- Hispanic—11.2%
- Non-Hispanic white—10.4%

*Adapted from MacDorman MF et al. *Pediatrics* 2002;110:1037-52

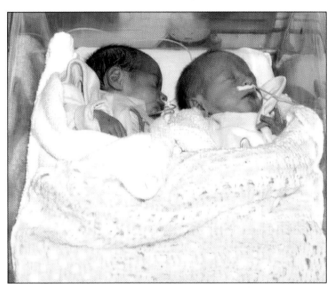

Twin pregnancy increases the risk of preterm birth

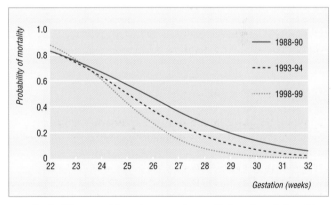

Mortality in UK neonatal intensive care cohorts of infants born before 32 weeks' gestation. Adapted from Parry G, et al. *Lancet* 2003;361:1789-91

Outcomes for infants live born before 26 weeks' gestation in British Isles*

Gestation (weeks)	Survival to discharge (%)	Survival without handicap at 30 months (%)
22	1	0.7
23	11	5
24	26	12
25	44	23

*Adapted from Wood NS et al. *New Engl J Med* 2000;343:378-84

improved outcome for preterm infants of multiple pregnancies has been attributed to closer surveillance of the mother and preterm obstetric intervention. As preterm multiple births are more likely to follow spontaneous preterm labour, the frequency of adverse factors—for example, severe intrauterine growth restriction, placental abruption, and fetomaternal infection—is lower than for preterm singletons.

Conclusion

The outcomes for preterm infants have improved greatly over the past 20-30 years in developed countries. Continued research is needed, however, to define the aetiology of preterm birth and identify interventions that will reduce its incidence.

Competing interests: WMcG received a grant from Pfizer UK for a national study of fungal infection in preterm infants.

The figure showing the definition of live births is adapted from Dunn PM, McIllwaine G, eds. *Perinatal audit: a report for the European Association of Perinatal Medicine*. London: Parthenon, 1996. The graph showing rates of preterm birth by gestational age group is adapted from Craig ED et al. *Arch Dis Child* 2002;86:142-6. The poster promoting smoking cessation in pregnancy is reproduced with permission from Group Against Smoking in Public, Bristol.

Further reading

- Slattery M, Morrison JJ. Preterm delivery. *Lancet* 2002;360:1489-97
- Kramer MS, Seguin L, Lydon, J, Goulet L. Socio-economic disparities in pregnancy outcome: why do the poor fare so poorly? *Paediatr Perinat Epidemiol* 2000;14:194-210
- Draper ES, Manktelow B, Field DJ, James D. Prediction of survival for preterm births by weight and gestational age: retrospective population based study. *BMJ* 1999;319:1093-7
- Wood NS, Marlow N, Costeloe K, Gibson AT, Wilkinson AR. Neurologic and developmental disability after extremely preterm birth. EPICure Study Group. *N Engl J Med* 2000;343:378-84
- Lumley J, Oliver S, Waters E. Interventions for promoting smoking cessation during pregnancy. *Cochrane Database Syst Rev* 2000;2:CD001055

2   Organisation and delivery of perinatal services

Janet Tucker, Gareth Parry, Peter W Fowlie, William McGuire

Over the past 30 years advances in antenatal and perinatal care have improved outcomes for preterm infants greatly. In the United Kingdom the neonatal mortality rate for very low birth weight infants (birth weight < 1500 g) fell from about 50% in 1975 to less than 20% in 1995. Additionally, the incidence of preterm stillbirth has fallen so that it seems that many more preterm infants are born alive than would have been the case 20-30 years ago.

With these advances in care comes a higher demand for perinatal services, particularly for intensive care for preterm infants. Services such as neonatal intensive care, however, have a low throughput of patients, use complex and technical equipment, and are expensive. Organising the delivery of these services is not simple.

Levels of care

The level of additional care that preterm infants need varies. Broadly, the level of care is inversely related to the gestational age and birth weight.
- Special care—for example, gastric tube feeding, temperature maintenance, and respiratory monitoring for apnoea
- High dependency care—for example, continuous monitoring, supplemental oxygen, and parenteral nutrition
- Intensive care—for example, mechanical ventilation, exogenous surfactant, and other organ support (such as the use of inotropes).

Most infants born after about 32 weeks of gestation or with a birth weight > 1500 g need special care only while they establish oral feeding and grow to sufficient maturity so that they can be safely discharged. Often the infant's mother is a major carer. Neonatal nurseries may have transitional care facilities to allow mothers to stay with their infants, particularly when they are establishing breast feeding.

Less mature (or less well) infants may need high dependency care for days or weeks before progressing to special care status. Commonly, these infants need supplemental oxygen treatment for mild respiratory distress syndrome or parenteral nutrition until enteral feeds are established.

Few preterm infants need intensive care. Those that do are mostly the 0.5% of infants who are born before 30-32 weeks' gestation. Often these infants need ventilatory support for respiratory distress syndrome or intensive haemodynamic monitoring and management. Intensive care for these infants is expensive, needing input from a skilled multidisciplinary team and costly facilities and equipment. These resources are limited.

A census of the neonatal intensive care units in the United Kingdom in 1996 found that one quarter lacked the recommended minimum of one medical specialist with prime responsibility for newborn infants. Nearly 80% of the intensive care units in the census did not have enough trained nurses.

Planning the service

The challenge for health service planners is to use scarce resources efficiently while making neonatal intensive care facilities widely accessible. The most common service model for achieving this balance is based upon networks of affiliated neonatal units serving a defined geographical region. In some places—for example, in North America and Australasia— formal

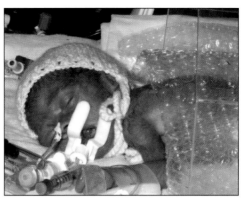
In intensive care preterm infants undergo mechanical ventilation

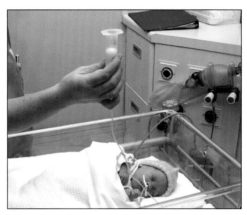
Infants in special care are often fed using a nasogastric tube containing maternal expressed breast milk

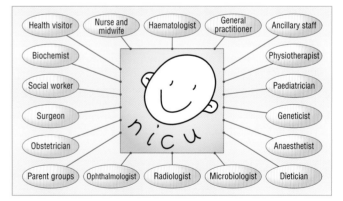
The multidisciplinary team contributes to infant and family centred care

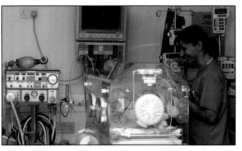
Limited resources in intensive care must be used efficiently

perinatal networks are well established. In others, such as the United Kingdom, there are formal regional networks and other groupings of more loosely affiliated units.

Units in the networks give a range of levels of care. Configurations of the networks vary according to local demography and geography. The regional neonatal intensive care units in rural and remote areas may serve a smaller population that is dispersed more widely than units in urban areas that are densely populated.

The aim of tiered networks of perinatal units is to ensure that the population in the region has local access to facilities that can at least provide special care. Fewer units in the region will provide high dependency care. In most regions, only one or two units will have the full range of medical intensive care services, although in the United Kingdom several smaller district hospitals in each region may provide intensive care. Centres that cover several regions usually have tertiary cardiology and surgical services.

Hospitals that can give only special care for newborn infants should arrange that preterm babies are delivered elsewhere. Mothers who will probably deliver early—for example, because of onset of spontaneous preterm labour or worsening maternal pre-eclampsia—should be transferred to the nearest unit in the network with high dependency or intensive care facilities.

Hospitals with only special care facilities must, however, have the equipment and appropriately trained staff for basic resuscitation and stabilisation of ill or very preterm infants unexpectedly born there. Robust mechanisms must be in place for the postnatal transfer of these infants to a unit with high dependency or intensive care services.

Transfers from regional centres

Regional neonatal intensive care units aim to work at near full capacity for most of the time so that expensive resources are not underused. However, demand for intensive care for preterm infants in individual units varies and is unpredictable. For example, preterm multiple birth can cause a sudden and unexpected increase in need for intensive care facilities. When a unit is already operating at or near to full capacity, mothers or preterm infants must sometimes be transferred to another unit for intensive care.

Unfortunately, such transfers from regional perinatal units often occur because of shortages of nursing staff. Mothers and infants may be transferred at short notice to a centre far from home. Such transfers are poor practice and undermine a family centred policy of care. The ongoing development of services for preterm infants and their families must deal with this issue.

Organisation and outcomes

The way that perinatal services are organised and delivered may have a substantial impact on important clinical outcomes, such as mortality or disability rates. Preterm infants who are cared for in the largest intensive care units, where staff can develop and maintain their skills, may have better outcomes than infants cared for in smaller, less busy units. In these large units, however, staff may become overworked and stressed so that mortality and morbidity of infants may increase. These considerations are central to the ongoing debate over whether intensive care services for preterm infants should be further centralised. In the United Kingdom, where neonatal intensive care units are often smaller than in other countries, this debate is especially relevant.

It is difficult to compare neonatal units (or health services) in different countries to determine if any differences in

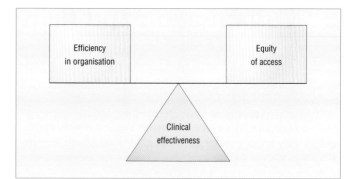

Planners try to achieve a balance between efficiency and accessibility to services

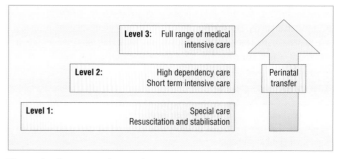

Neonatal units can provide varying levels of care. The tiered perinatal care network allows the population in the region to at least have access to special care facilities locally

---

Recommendations of the British Association of Perinatal Medicine for essential resuscitation and stabilisation

- Incubator care
- Monitoring of vital signs
- Venous access—fluids and drug administration
- Artificial ventilation
- Portable x ray facilities
- Drainage of a pneumothorax
- Administration of surfactant

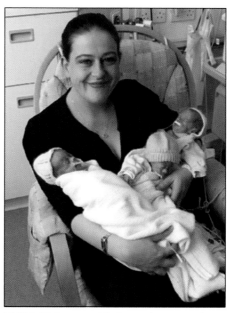

Multiple births can suddenly stretch resources in neonatal intensive care units

outcomes are caused by the way care is given rather than other factors. Larger perinatal centres care for a higher proportion of smaller and less mature infants, and these infants will have a higher risk of adverse outcomes because of the severity of their illness at birth. Using a validated risk adjustment tool, such as the clinical risk index for babies II, makes comparisons between centres fairer.

The United Kingdom Neonatal Staffing Study used a risk adjustment tool to determine if size of neonatal unit, staffing level, and unit workload had an effect on mortality and disability rates for infants that were admitted to neonatal intensive care. The study found that clinical networks seemed to be operating adequately, with the sickest infants often being cared for in larger units. After risk adjustment, mortality and morbidity outcomes were similar in large, medium, and low volume units. However, nearly all units cared for more infants than their recommended capacity at some point during the study. Importantly, evidence showed that infants who were admitted when neonatal intensive care units were getting busier had a significantly greater risk of dying. This evidence supports the idea that the overall performance of staff in intensive care units deteriorates as workload rises.

Conclusion

Perinatal health services must use limited resources efficiently to optimise the delivery of care for preterm infants and their families. This balance can be achieved by giving different levels of care in tiered clinical networks of neonatal units that serve a defined geographical area. Demands for professionals who provide neonatal intensive care to become more specialised indicate that there will be continued pressure towards centralisation of these services.

This centralisation may exacerbate the adverse workload effect seen in busier units. Additionally, centralised services would be especially difficult for families whose preterm infants need several weeks of care in a centre far from home. Before the configuration of specialist services for preterm infants is altered, associated maternity services and the acceptability of the changes to the parents and families of preterm infants for whom the service works must be considered.

The line drawing showing the tiered perinatal care network is adapted from material from the British Association of Perinatal Medicine. The photograph of a woman with triplets is reproduced with permission of the *Courier* (Dundee). The figures showing risk of death for infants in high, medium, and low volume neonatal intensive care units in the United Kingdom and risk of death for infants in neonatal units according to occupancy of unit on admission are adapted from Tucker J. *Lancet* 2002;359:99-107.

Components of the clinical risk index for babies II

- Sex
- Birth weight
- Gestation
- Base excess
- Temperature on admission to neonatal unit

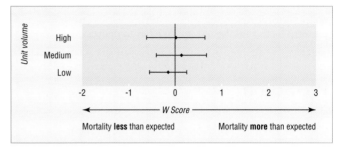

Risk of death for infants in high, medium, and low volume neonatal intensive care units in the United Kingdom

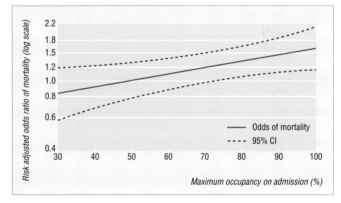

Risk of death for infants in neonatal units according to occupancy of unit on admission

Further reading

- Clinical Standards Advisory Group (CSAG). *Access to and availability of specialist services.* London: HMSO, 1993
- Parry G, Tucker J, Tarnow-Mordi W. CRIB II: updating the clinical risk index for babies (CRIB) score using a representative UK sample of infants admitted for neonatal intensive care. *Lancet* 2003;361:1789-91
- Tucker J. UK Neonatal Staffing Study Group: a prospective evaluation of patient volume, staffing and workload in relation to risk-adjusted outcomes in a random, stratified sample of all UK neonatal intensive care units. *Lancet* 2002;359:99-107

3 Obstetric issues in preterm birth

Deirdre J Murphy, Peter W Fowlie, William McGuire

Predicting and preventing preterm labour and choosing the safest method of delivery are important challenges in reducing the number of preterm births and improving outcomes for mother and baby. This article covers the predictive tests, methods of prevention, maternal and fetal indications for preterm birth, and various approaches to delivery.

Prediction

Most preterm deliveries follow spontaneous onset of preterm labour or preterm prelabour rupture of the amniotic membranes (pPROM). Much work has been done (with limited success) to find diagnostic tests that predict accurately if a woman who is at risk of preterm delivery will go on to deliver preterm. For these women, who may have a history of preterm birth or clinical signs of preterm labour, such tests would allow early and targeted use of antenatal interventions. These interventions, especially antenatal corticosteroids, improve neonatal and long term outcomes for preterm infants.

The most common clinical tests used to determine the risk of preterm labour are transvaginal sonography (to measure the length of the endocervix) and the cervicovaginal fetal fibronectin test. These tests have high negative predictive values—that is, if results are negative then the women probably will not progress to preterm delivery. Although there does not seem to be a role for routine use of the fibronectin test or transvaginal sonography to screen women for preterm birth, women thought to be at high risk can be reassured by negative results. This may help women to avoid unnecessary interventions such as antenatal transfer to a distant perinatal unit.

Prevention

Current medical approaches to preventing preterm labour include the use of tocolytic drugs, antibiotic treatment, and cervical cerclage.

Tocolytic drugs
Tocolytic drugs can delay the progress of preterm labour in the short term but maternal side effects include hypotension, tachycardia, and fluid overload. No evidence exists to show that tocolysis improves perinatal outcomes; however, the delay in delivery may allow enough time to give the woman antenatal steroids or to arrange her transfer to a perinatal centre with neonatal intensive care facilities if needed.

Antibiotic treatment
The recent ORACLE II trial concluded that antibiotics should not be prescribed routinely for women in preterm labour who have intact fetal membranes and no evidence of clinical infection.

A systematic review of randomised controlled trials (including the large ORACLE I trial) indicated that antibiotics for preterm prelabour membrane rupture prolong pregnancy and reduce the incidence of neonatal infection. Antibiotic prophylaxis, however, is not associated with a substantial

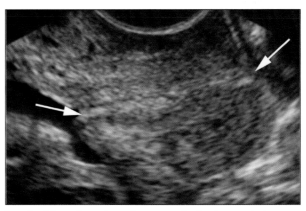

Length of the endocervix can be measured using transvaginal sonography

---

Antenatal corticosteroids

- Reduce perinatal mortality, respiratory distress syndrome, and intraventricular haemorrhage
- Have maximum benefit when delivery occurs 24 hours to seven days after treatment
- When fetus remains undelivered repeated courses have uncertain benefit

---

Cervicovaginal fetal fibronectin test

Fibronectin is:
- Glycoprotein in amniotic fluid or placental tissue
- Released because of damage to membrane of placenta
- Measured from cervical or vaginal swabs

Tocolytic drugs

- β_2 agonists
- Calcium channel blockers
- Prostaglandin synthetase inhibitors
- Magnesium sulphate
- Oxytocin antagonists

When fetal membranes are intact, with no signs of clinical infection, antibiotics do not seem to prolong pregnancy or improve neonatal health

reduction in perinatal mortality. Long term follow up data from ORACLE I will show if antibiotic prophylaxis affects neurodevelopmental impairment in preterm infants born after prelabour membrane rupture.

Cervical cerclage
Reports conflict over the value of prophylactic, therapeutic, or rescue cervical cerclage for women at risk of preterm labour because of cervical incompetence. A systematic review indicates that this invasive procedure should be considered only for women at very high risk of miscarriage in the second trimester or extremely preterm labour. Identifying these women is not easy. Further large randomised controlled trials are needed.

Screening for bacterial vaginosis
Bacterial vaginosis is overgrowth of anaerobic bacteria in the vagina. It can predispose women to preterm delivery. Current evidence does not support screening and treating asymptomatic pregnant women for bacterial vaginosis. For women with a history of preterm birth, detecting and treating bacterial vaginosis early in pregnancy may prevent a proportion of these women having a further preterm birth.

Maternal and fetal indications

About 15% to 25% of preterm births are caused by obstetric or medical complications of pregnancy. Obstetric complications such as pre-eclampsia may result in maternal morbidity or mortality and perinatal death if the infant is not delivered. Maternal risks of pre-eclampsia include eclamptic seizures, cerebral haemorrhage, HELLP (haemolysis, elevated liver enzymes, low platelets) syndrome, and maternal death.

Women with diabetes, renal disease, autoimmune disease, and congenital heart disease need intensive surveillance. Preterm delivery may be indicated because of deterioration of maternal or fetal health, and obstetric complications may occur.

When planning the timing and mode of delivery of preterm infants in these circumstances, it is necessary to weigh the risks to the mother and fetus of continuing the pregnancy against the risks of preterm birth and delivery. With the potentially compromised very preterm fetus, the aim is to allow the pregnancy to continue to a point before damage occurs without taking unnecessary risks that may harm the mother.

Several tests of fetal wellbeing are available. In high risk pregnancies, fetal growth is usually monitored using serial ultrasonography to measure circumference of the head and abdominal girth. A fall in the growth velocity of the abdominal circumference indicates intrauterine growth restriction.

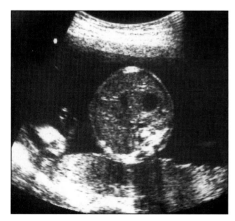

Abdominal circumference shown on ultrasonography is used to assess fetal growth

Cervical cerclage is circumferential suturing around the cervical os

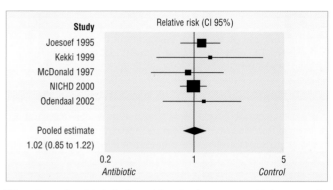

Effect of use of antibiotic for bacterial vaginosis on preterm birth compared with placebo. Adapted from Macdonald H et al. *Cochrane Database Syst Rev* 2003;2:CD000262

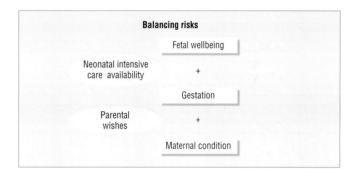

Many factors must be taken into account when deciding the timing and type of delivery

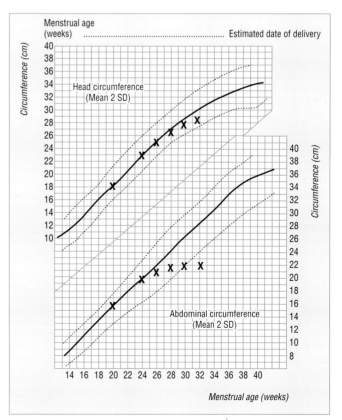

Growth charts are used to plot the circumference of the head and abdomen over time (menstrual weeks). This chart shows the progress of a fetus with intrauterine growth restriction

Cardiotocography and fetal biophysical profiling are two tools often used to determine the physiological status of the potentially compromised fetus. Unfortunately these tools have no benefit in predicting and preventing poor outcomes in high risk pregnancies. Some evidence shows, however, that computerised cardiotocography is more accurate in predicting poor outcome than subjective clinical assessment alone. The biophysical profile takes into account the tone, movement, breathing, heart rate pattern of the fetus, and liquor volume.

Doppler

Umbilical arterial blood flow becomes abnormal when there is placental insufficiency—for example, secondary to pre-eclampsia. Doppler measurement of fetoplacental blood velocity may be a more useful test of fetal wellbeing than cardiocotography or biophysical profiling. However, a recent systematic review of randomised controlled trials did not indicate that Doppler measurement of fetoplacental blood velocity is associated with a substantial reduction in perinatal mortality. Additionally, there is uncertainty over the ideal frequency of examination and the optimum threshold for intervention. Umbilical artery Doppler ultrasonography to detect fetal compromise is part of routine obstetric practice for high risk pregnancies in many countries, so there may not be further randomised controlled trials in high risk populations.

Recent studies have investigated the use of middle cerebral artery and ductus venosus Doppler waveforms in evaluating cardiovascular adaptations to placental insufficiency. Results are promising, although the effect on important outcomes when used as part of clinical practice has yet to be evaluated.

Preventing pre-eclampsia

Women who have had pre-eclampsia can be given low doses of aspirin in a future pregnancy. In a systematic review of randomised trials that involved over 30 000 women, prophylactic antiplatelet treatment that was started in the first trimester reduced the risk of recurrent pre-eclampsia and stillbirth and neonatal death by about 15%.

Calcium supplements in the diet can reduce the risk of hypertension and pre-eclampsia associated with pregnancy for women at high risk, and in communities with a low intake of dietary calcium.

Mode of delivery

Vaginal delivery of the preterm infant is associated with lower maternal morbidity than delivery by caesarean section. It is important, however, to consider the following points:
● Obstetric history
● Likely interval between induction and delivery in the context of deterioration of maternal health
● Probability of achieving a vaginal delivery versus risk of emergency caesarean section
● Presentation and prelabour condition of the fetus.

Breech delivery

In developed countries with good antenatal services most term breech pregnancies are managed by elective caesarean section, as are many multiple pregnancies. The increase in caesarean sections has caused a loss of obstetric skill in vaginal delivery of breech and multiple pregnancies. Most planned preterm breech and twin pregnancies are delivered by elective caesarean section even though there is no clear evidence of benefit.

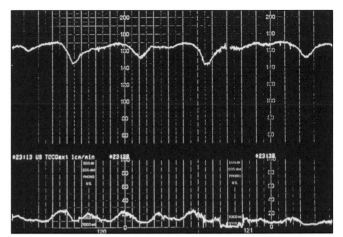

Monitoring the fetal heart rate can help determine the physiological wellbeing of the fetus. This cardiotocogram shows fetal tachycardia with reduced variability and decelerations

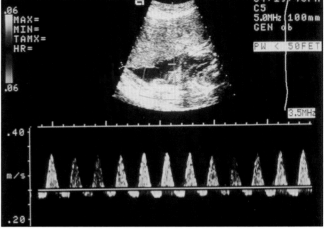

Doppler measurement of umbilical arterial flow is used to test fetal wellbeing. This recording shows reversed end diastolic velocity waveform

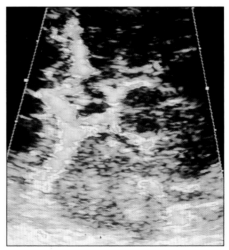

Doppler measurement of middle cerebral arterial flow. Abnormal waveforms can show cardiovascular adaptations to placental insufficiency

Induction of labour is most likely to be successful in a woman with a favourable cervix (as assessed by the Bishop score) who has had no caesarean sections and has a history of vaginal delivery

Extremely preterm birth

When planning preterm delivery before 26 weeks' gestation, it is important to consider the overall reproductive outcome for the mother. The choice of the most appropriate mode of delivery for extremely preterm infants is affected by the difficulty in carrying out a lower segment caesarean section at such early gestations and the potential for substantial fetal trauma. Classic (vertical incision) caesarean section presents major risks for the mother. After classic caesarean section, elective caesarean section for subsequent pregnancies is mandatory because there is an increased risk of uterine rupture and perinatal death. These issues are difficult for prospective parents and any discussion is limited by a lack of robust evidence to guide practice.

Conclusion

Predicting and preventing preterm labour remain elusive goals. Greater numbers of preterm deliveries are planned because of early recognition of obstetric complications, an increase in women who plan pregnancies in the context of medical disorders, and a lowering in the threshold for viability. The aim in these circumstances is to achieve a timely delivery by the safest route possible. Advances in neonatal care have improved perinatal outcome considerably, but the falling threshold of viability has created a new set of dilemmas for parents and carers.

Further reading

- Crowley P. Prophylactic corticosteroids for preterm birth. *Cochrane Database Syst Rev* 2003;(4):CD000065
- Honest H, Bachmann LM, Gupta JK, Kleijnen J, Khan KS. Accuracy of cervicovaginal fetal fibronectin test in predicting spontaneous preterm birth: systematic review. *BMJ* 2002;325:301-4
- King J, Flenady V. Prophylactic antibiotics for inhibiting preterm labour with intact membranes. *Cochrane Database Syst Rev* 2003;(4):CD000246
- Kenyon S, Boulvain M, Neilson J. Antibiotics for preterm rupture of membranes. *Cochrane Database Syst Rev* 2003;(4):CD001058
- Knight M, Duley L, Henderson-Smart DJ, King JF. Antiplatelet agents for preventing and treating pre-eclampsia. *Cochrane Database Syst Rev* 2003;(4):CD000492
- Hofmeyr GJ, Atallah AN, Duley L. Calcium supplementation during pregnancy for preventing hypertensive disorders and related problems. *Cochrane Database Syst Rev* 2003;(4):CD001059
- Neilson JP, Alfirevic Z. Doppler ultrasound for fetal assessment in high risk pregnancies. *Cochrane Database Syst Rev* 2003;(4):CD000073

Competing interests: DJM has provided expert opinion on preterm birth in medicolegal cases.

The photograph of transvaginal sonography measuring cervical length is courtesy of the Fetal Medicine Foundation, London, and the remaining images are courtesy of Professor Phillipa Kyle.

4 Immediate care of the preterm infant

Peter W Fowlie, William McGuire

Preparing appropriately for the delivery and immediate care of the preterm infant is essential when time permits and may impact on the eventual outcome for the infant. This article describes the skills and equipment needed for the care and possible resuscitation of these vulnerable babies. The support and advice needed by parents and families at this time is also explored.

Preparation for preterm delivery

When preterm delivery can be anticipated there may be an opportunity for paediatric staff to discuss intrapartum and postnatal care with prospective parents and colleagues from midwifery and obstetrics. Even if detailed discussion is not possible, relevant historical details should be taken to anticipate problems and prepare appropriately for the arrival of the preterm infant.

Broadly, the level of resuscitation that may be needed is inversely related to the gestation of the preterm infant. Usually, the approach taken in resuscitating preterm infants of > 32 completed weeks' gestation is the same as that taken for term infants. Most need only basic measures such as drying and stimulation. Infants of gestation < 32 weeks (or birth weight < 1500 g) require more active support. For infants of < 28 weeks' gestation, this support will probably include endotracheal intubation and assisted ventilation.

Ideally, two members of staff who are experienced in the early care of preterm infants should be present at the delivery of each anticipated infant. A senior paediatrician with extensive experience in dealing with preterm babies should be at the delivery of infants of < 28 weeks' gestation. Before delivery, the attending staff should recheck essential equipment for resuscitation.

Equipment for resuscitation of the preterm infant

- Clock with second hand
- Dry, warmed towels and heat source
- Light source
- Wide bore suction device
- Facemasks in a variety of sizes
- Inflatable bag with blow-off valve
- Oxygen source with pressure limiting device
- Laryngoscope with neonatal blades
- Endotracheal tube (sizes 2.5, 3.0, and 3.5)
- Needles and syringes
- Umbilical catheters

Assessment and resuscitation

Preterm infants get cold quickly because of their relatively large surface area. Resulting hypothermia reduces surfactant production, may hasten hypoglycaemia and acidaemia, and is associated with increased mortality. Preterm infants should be delivered into warm towels, dried, and transferred to a dedicated neonatal resuscitation platform or trolley with an integral radiant heater. Alternatively, immediate occlusive wrapping in polythene may be at least as effective in reducing evaporative heat loss, especially in extremely preterm infants.

History relevant to preterm delivery

- Maternal medical and obstetric history
- Estimated gestation
- Singleton or multifetal pregnancy?
- Assessments of fetal growth and wellbeing
- Details of suspected congenital anomalies
- Risk of fetal-maternal infection and chorioamnionitis
- Course of labour, if labouring
- Intrapartum monitoring results
- Antenatal interventions, tocolytic drugs, steroids, antibiotics
- Use of opiates and anaesthetic drugs

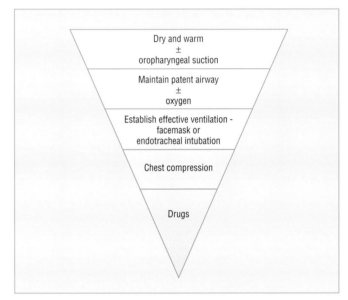

The "inverted triangle" shows how commonly certain interventions are needed

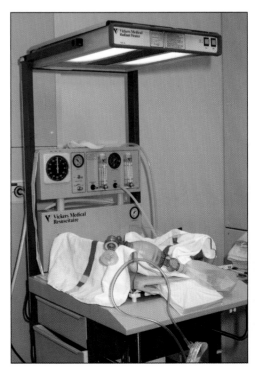

Preterm infants should be moved to a neonatal resuscitation trolley with radiant heater after delivery as they get cold quickly

As with all acute resuscitation, the aims are to ensure airway patency and support the breathing and circulation. Colour, respiratory effort, tone, and heart rate can be assessed to determine the response of the infant to interventions.

Airway
To obtain a patent airway, the infant's head should be maintained in a neutral position and the chin should be supported while applying gentle forward traction to the mandible (jaw thrust). Careful suction under direct vision may be used to clear secretions that can obstruct the airway.

Breathing
Failure to establish regular breathing in the first minute after birth is an indication for assisted ventilation. The aim is to inflate the newborn's poorly compliant, fluid filled lungs to recruit alveoli for gas exchange. About five initial "inflation" breaths of 2-3 seconds' duration followed by ventilation at a rate of around 40 breaths per minute using pressures of 20-25 cm H_2O is appropriate while checking for spontaneous respiration every 30 seconds. Occasionally, higher inflation pressures, up to 30 cm H_2O, may be needed. The benefit of using positive end expiratory pressure as part of acute resuscitation has yet to be established. Commonly, 100% oxygen is used, but no evidence exists that this achieves better outcomes than lower concentrations of oxygen.

Inflation breaths, and subsequent ventilation if spontaneous respiration is not established, can be delivered via a facemask attached to a Y piece system with a blow-off valve or via a bag valve mask. A range of masks should be available to fit over the infant's mouth and nose (but not the orbital margin). Staff caring for newborn infants in all centres, including community maternity units, should be trained to deliver facemask ventilation effectively.

Infants of >32 weeks' gestation
For infants of gestation > 32 weeks, failure to respond to appropriately delivered facemask ventilation in the first 2-3 minutes is rare, and may be an indication for endotracheal intubation.

Infants of 28-32 weeks' gestation
Infants born at < 32 weeks' gestation have an increased risk of surfactant deficiency and of developing respiratory distress syndrome. In addition, they have less developed respiratory muscles than term infants and are less able to cope with the increased work of breathing associated with poorly compliant lungs.

For infants of gestation 28-32 weeks who do not establish adequate spontaneous respiration in 30-60 seconds, other options to sustain respiration exist. These options include supporting ventilation with continuous positive airway pressure via nasal prongs or facemask, intubating and providing intermittent positive pressure ventilation, and administering prophylactic surfactant.

Infants of < 28 weeks' gestation
Not all infants of < 28 weeks' gestation need intubation at birth. Unless the infant is pink and active, however, immediate endotracheal intubation at birth should be considered. In these infants there is evidence that early prophylactic replacement of natural surfactant is more effective than delayed "rescue" treatment in reducing the incidence of acute lung injury and mortality. For infants born outside the labour ward, resuscitative efforts should concentrate on keeping the infant warm, maintaining a clear airway, administering oxygen, and applying facemask ventilation.

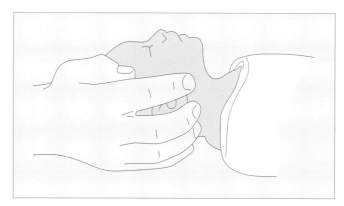
Correct head position for newborn resuscitation—the neutral position

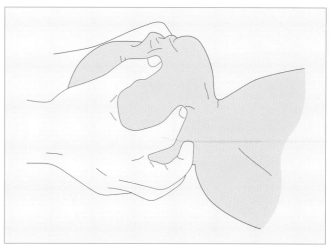
Jaw thrust for maintaining a patent airway in newborn infant

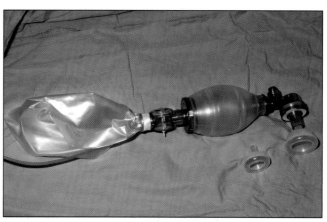
Bag valve mask can be used to deliver inflation breaths and subsequent ventilation if necessary

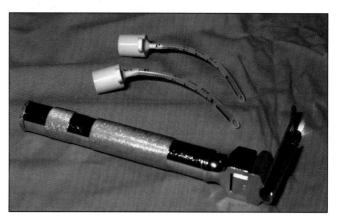
Laryngoscope and endotracheal tubes for intubating preterm infants

Circulation

Chest compression is indicated if, despite adequate artificial ventilation, the infant's heart rate remains < 60 beats per minute and is not improving. Apply around 90 compressions per minute with lung reinflation after every three chest compressions.

Drugs

If there is no improvement in clinical condition after adequate ventilation and chest compression, then certain drugs may be useful in the acute resuscitation of preterm infants. Persistent bradycardia may respond to adrenaline (epinephrine) and sometimes intravenous sodium bicarbonate can be used to correct acidosis. Dextrose may also be useful during prolonged resuscitation to correct hypoglycaemia. The use of intravenous fluids (normal saline, plasma, and blood) for volume expansion in preterm infants should be limited to those infants known to have volume depletion—for example, after antepartum haemorrhage.

All drugs are best delivered via an umbilical venous catheter. Adrenaline (epinephrine) may be given via the endotracheal route although its efficacy is unknown when given this way. Sadly, infants who do not respond to appropriate "basic" resuscitation and merit drug intervention will probably have a poor prognosis.

Stopping intensive resuscitation efforts

If the heart rate does not improve despite 15-20 minutes of appropriate efforts, then it may be appropriate to stop resuscitation and to provide palliative care. A decision to stop active intervention should be made by senior staff in consultation with the parents. If an experienced member of staff is not available resuscitation should be continued until a senior colleague is contacted.

Infants born at the threshold of viability

Although interventions (such as prophylactic antenatal steroids and exogenous surfactants) have improved certain outcomes for extremely preterm infants, recent data indicate that the overall prognosis for infants born at < 26 weeks' gestation remains poor. When delivery at < 26 weeks' gestation is anticipated, the most experienced paediatrician available must counsel the parents and inform them of the potential outcomes for mother and infant.

If possible, the parents should then be allowed to reflect on the implications of this information before it is decided how to care for the newborn infant. Some parents and carers may feel that aggressive perinatal interventions are not in the best interests of the infant and family. Such discussions and any decisions reached should be documented and conveyed to all staff who are caring for the mother or infant. The parents should be assured that any decision to withhold or start resuscitation can be revised at any time depending on clinical circumstances.

Palliative care of the newborn infant

If resuscitation is unsuccessful, or if active resuscitation is felt to be inappropriate, then palliative care should be provided for the infant and family. The parents can spend time with their baby,

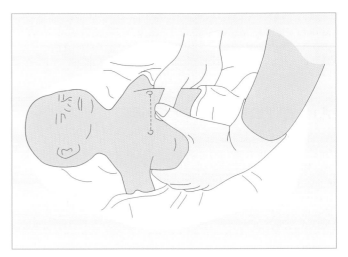

Chest compressions may be needed to resuscitate newborns if their heart rates are <60 beats per minute and there is no improvement in response to respiratory support

---

Drugs used in acute resuscitation of the preterm infant

- Adrenaline (epinephrine) (1:10 000): 0.1 ml/kg (10 μg/kg)
- Sodium bicarbonate (4.2%): 2-4 ml/kg (1-2 mmol/kg)
- Dextrose (10%): 2.5 ml/kg (250 mg/kg)
- Intravenous volume replacement: saline (0.9%), plasma, blood: 10-20 ml/kg

All given via an umbilical venous catheter; adrenaline may also be given via endotracheal tube.

Perinatal management at the threshold of viability

- Antenatal counselling should be provided by senior neonatologists, obstetricians, and midwives
- Management decisions should depend on what the parents and their medical advisers think is in the child's best interests
- Parents should have accurate information on likely outcomes for their infant—including their chances of survival and the risk of longer term disability
- Information on outcomes provided to parents should cite data from large cohort studies that reported the outcome of all pregnancies for each week of gestation (not just for infants admitted to intensive care units)
- Perinatal management plans should consider the mode of delivery, use of intrapartum monitoring, and immediate care of the newborn
- Decisions not to provide active resuscitation or intensive care should not be binding, particularly if the newborn seems more mature than anticipated
- It may be appropriate to provide full resuscitation and intensive care to infants at birth until the clinical progress becomes clearer and further discussions with the family have been possible
- Parents should be supported throughout and encouraged to seek advice and further support from others, such as family members and religious advisers
- Infants who are not actively resuscitated or in whom active resuscitation is withdrawn should receive palliative care

---

Factors needed in the palliative care of extremely preterm infants

- Warmth
- Dignity
- Human contact
- Pain relief

and should be aware that their baby may show signs of life, such as occasional gasps, after birth. Privacy and sensitive support for parents and family with subsequent follow up are essential. The potential importance of postmortem examination should be discussed at an appropriate time.

Audit and review

All deliveries of extremely preterm infants should be reviewed by the neonatal service as part of training and good practice. Particular attention should be given to aspects of care that have been shown to affect outcome. Regular perinatal meetings are an ideal opportunity to examine these episodes of care and should be mandatory for any neonatal service.

The line drawings of head position, jaw thrust and chest compressions in newborns are adapted from *Resuscitation at birth: newborn life support provider course manual.* London: Resuscitation Council (UK), 2001. The box on perinatal management at the threshold of viability is adapted from the British Association of Perinatal Medicine practice framework (www.bapm.org/documents/publications/)

Further reading

- Joint Working Party of Royal College of Paediatrics and Child Health and Royal College of Obstetricians and Gynaecologists. *Resuscitation of babies at birth.* London: BMJ Publishing Group, 1997
- Wood NS, Marlow N, Costeloe K, Gibson AT, Wilkinson AR. Neurologic and developmental disability after extremely preterm birth. EPICure Study Group. *N Engl J Med* 2000;343:378-84
- Gee H, Dunn P. Fetuses and newborn infants at the threshold of viability: a framework for practice. *Perinat Neonat Med* 2000;5:209-11
- Resuscitation Council (UK). *Resuscitation at birth: newborn life support provider course manual.* London: Resuscitation Council (UK), 2002
- Soll RF, Morley CJ. Prophylactic versus selective use of surfactant in preventing morbidity and mortality in preterm infants. *Cochrane Database Syst Rev* 2003;(3):CD000510

5 Moving the preterm infant

Peter W Fowlie, Philip Booth, Charles H Skeoch

Many different health service models for providing neonatal intensive care have been established over the past 30 years, and much of the developed world is moving towards a centralised model of care. At least initially, preterm infants often require specialised care in an intensive care setting. As a result, newborn infants and pregnant mothers may have to move between hospitals for appropriate care because of prematurity or the threat of preterm delivery. Sometimes this move means that the infant and family have to travel hundreds of miles.

This article focuses on the postnatal transfer of preterm infants between hospitals. Antenatal transfer of pregnant women is not considered here, although in utero transfer has better clinical outcomes for mother and infant than transfer after birth. Many of the issues discussed are applicable to transfers within hospitals.

Interhospital transport services

In utero transfer is not always possible—for example, if labour is too advanced. Of the several models for transporting newborn infants, the most sophisticated are regional transport services that carry out all neonatal moves in a defined area using dedicated staff and equipment. These teams are responsible for neonatal transport only and are often "independent," not being affiliated to a particular maternity or neonatal unit. A medical director usually runs such regional services, and the staff carrying out the transports may be medical or nursing staff with other professionals sometimes contributing. Referring hospitals and receiving hospitals do not have to provide staff or equipment, and each transport is undertaken by dedicated staff who have training and experience in transporting sick neonates.

When no regional transport service is available, medical and nursing staff from either referring or receiving units undertake the transport on an ad hoc basis. The staff will have variable experience in neonatal transport and the equipment used, and the vehicle may not be dedicated for neonatal use. Running these ad hoc teams often puts resources under strain because there will be fewer staff on site in the unit that carries out the transport. With less experienced staff, the risk of adverse events on such transports can be greater than with dedicated teams. In some parts of the world even ad hoc transport services are not available and transports with no clinical escort or untrained escorts use unsuitable equipment and vehicles.

Safe transport of the preterm infant

Anticipating the need for transfer early, appropriate preparation for transfer, and ongoing high quality care during transfer, are the cornerstones of good neonatal transport. To achieve this staff need to be trained appropriately, all equipment and vehicles must be fit for the purpose, and lines of communication must be well established.

Anticipation
When in utero transfer is not possible, there may still be an opportunity to seek advice, gather staff with the right skills, and prepare appropriate equipment. Direct communication between senior staff in the two centres involved is important.

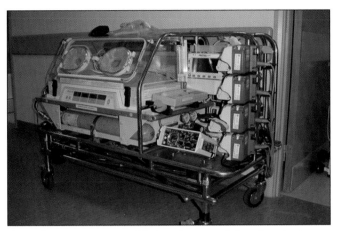

Neonatal transport system—mobile intensive care unit for safe and comfortable transport of infants

---

Reasons for transferring preterm infants between hospitals

- No appropriate local neonatal facilities
- No cots available locally (neonatal intensive care unit or special care baby unit "full")
- Insufficient appropriate nursing or medical staff available locally—for example, paediatric surgeons, cardiologists
- Unexpected delivery far from home
- Transfers back to local facility

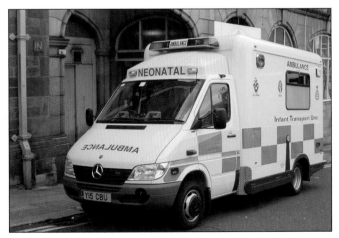

An ambulance dedicated to, and equipped for, neonatal transport

The ethos of neonatal transport medicine is to keep the infant stable and, preferably, improve the clinical status of the infant

Stabilisation

Preparing for transport begins as soon as the decision to move an infant is made. Specific treatments such as antibiotic treatment, surfactant replacement, volume support or inotrope support, analgesia, sedation, paralysis, anticonvulsant treatment, and nitric oxide should be considered. Any remedial action should be taken before moving the baby and not during the transport. Although the infant should be in as good a clinical condition as possible before setting off, the decision to stabilise the infant further or institute specific treatments must be weighed against a delay in transfer. These difficult decisions should be made in collaboration with experienced staff. The choices made will depend on many factors, including the clinical condition and progress of the infant, experience of staff on site, and equipment and treatments available.

Infant care during the journey

With good preparation and stabilisation before setting off, minimal active intervention should be needed during the transfer. However, infants can deteriorate spontaneously (for example, pneumothorax), or equipment (for example, endotracheal tubes and intravenous lines) can be dislodged. Equipment to deal with such eventualities must be carried.

The infant's temperature should be maintained during any journey. When possible, the environmental temperature of the vehicle should be raised.

Communication and documentation

Good verbal and written communication between health professionals throughout transport episodes is vital. Using clinical guidelines, operational policies, and checklists is helpful. Parents also need to know plans for their baby's care, and the transport team should meet the parents when possible. In some settings informed consent is needed for transport and care. If parents are not travelling in the ambulance with their infant, they may need to know how to get to the destination hospital and what facilities will be available for them when they arrive. Helpful written information (for example, leaflets about the destination neonatal unit and maps) can be stored electronically and downloaded as needed.

Choice of vehicle

Different types of vehicles can be used to transport neonates. The mode of transport that is most appropriate will depend on resource availability, geography, clinical pathology, urgency of the situation, and the experience of the staff. More organisation is needed for an air transfer than for road transfers. Air transfer also requires specialist training and skills from staff, and the important physiological effects of flying must be taken into account. These effects include hypoxia, barometric pressure drop, thermal change, dehydration, gravitational forces, noise, vibration, and fatigue.

Equipment

Systems are based around an incubator fixed to a transport trolley with integrated ventilator, monitor, intravenous pump, and medical gas supply. Unfortunately, an infant cannot be secured in the transport incubator itself, and so is susceptible to substantial movement and potential trauma if there is sudden movement. Comfort factors (such as warmth, noise reduction, padding, and chemical sedation) can be adjusted.

The equipment should be designed to function while in motion. Although adequate portable power sources should be available, all equipment should be run from the transport vehicle's power supply if possible. Medical gases sourced from the transport vehicle should be used whenever possible.

Clinical stabilisation before transfer

Airway
- Is the airway patent?
- Is the airway secure?

Breathing
- Is the infant making sufficient spontaneous respiratory effort?
- If not, is artificial ventilation adequate?

Circulation
- Are the baby's essential organs perfusing adequately?

Metabolic
- Is the baby's blood glucose adequate?
- Is the baby's acid-base balance acceptable?

Temperature control
- Is the baby's temperature normal?
- Is the baby in a thermoneutral environment?

Comfort
- Is the baby being exposed to any noxious stimuli?
- Does the baby need chemical sedation?

Minimising heat loss from the infant during transport
- Raise the environmental temperature of the vehicle if possible
- Ensure doors of vehicle are closed
- Ensure doors of transport incubator are closed
- Use a heated gel mattress (also helps absorb vibration and improve general comfort for the infant)

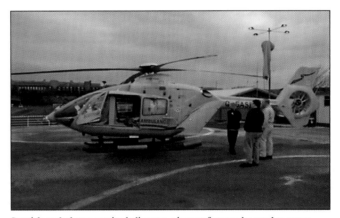

Scottish ambulance service helicopter—air transfer may be used to move infants depending on factors such as the geography of the journey, urgency of the situation, and the experience of the available staff

---

Transport equipment*
- Transport incubator mounted on appropriate trolley
- Monitors for heart rate, respiratory rate, temperature, blood pressure (invasive and non-invasive), inspired oxygen concentration, oxygen saturation, and end tidal carbon dioxide
- Assisted ventilation equipment
- Suction apparatus
- Equipment for intubation, intravascular infusion (central or peripheral, venous or arterial), chest tube placement
- Drugs
- Portable blood gas analyser
- Portable blood glucose analyser
- Medical gases (oxygen, air, and nitric oxide)

*This list is not all-inclusive, and equipment taken on neonatal transport must be appropriate for the clinical situation and the likely journey

Estimates for the quantity of all medical gases needed should allow for delays. Gas consumption can be estimated as flow delivered (l/min) × fraction of inspired oxygen × journey time (minutes) × 2.

Many types of equipment bag exist and their contents vary, depending on the type of move. Bearing in mind that too much can cause confusion in an emergency, equipment should be kept to the minimum required for essential procedures.

Staff safety

Transport systems should comply with regulations on the safe loading and fixation of transport incubators in vehicles. Staff may sustain serious injury if loose equipment is dislodged during a journey, or while loading the transport systems. Historically, transport systems have been extremely heavy, sometimes over 200 kg, although lighter systems have now been developed. In the United Kingdom the health and safety regulation limit is 140 kg. The transport system must be fixed securely in the vehicle using a mechanism that has been appropriately "crash tested." All employers should have adequate insurance that covers staff and equipment.

Personnel and training

Transporting sick preterm infants requires specific skills and a high level of clinical competence. All staff involved—medical, nursing, paramedical, and others such as medical physicists—should have appropriate training in neonatal transport medicine, be familiar with local organisational procedures, and know how to use the equipment. No agreed standards on training in neonatal transport medicine exist in the United Kingdom. However, formal training programmes are becoming available.

Risk management

Clinical risk management aims to identify shortfalls in standards and suggest appropriate remedial action. Unfortunately, only broad national clinical standards are available. However, some specific standards against which transport services can be audited have been used locally. Non-clinical aspects of neonatal transport medicine can be audited against directives from the Health and Safety Executive and medical electrical equipment standards. Audit and review with regard to avoidable adverse events is vital to the ongoing improvement and development of transport services for preterm infants.

Conclusion

Some newborn infants will always need to be moved between hospitals. Neonatal transport services must be well organised and should aim to provide clinical care to a high standard. The service should be staffed by professionals trained in neonatal transport medicine and in using appropriate equipment.

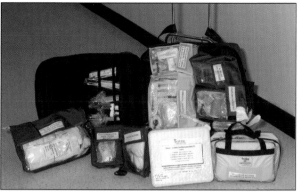

Equipment bags and their contents vary according to the type of neonatal transport that they are used for

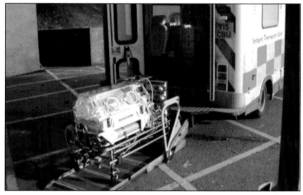

Loading mechanism for loading transport incubators into ambulances. All transport systems must meet regulation standards

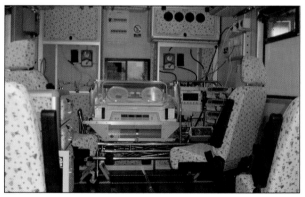

Neonatal transport unit must be secured safely in the ambulance

Further reading

- British Association of Perinatal Medicine. *Standards for hospitals providing neonatal intensive care.* 2nd ed. London: British Association of Perinatal Medicine, 2001
- Schlossman PA, Manley JS, Sciscione AC, Colmorgen GH. An analysis of neonatal morbidity and mortality in maternal (in utero) and neonatal transports at 24-34 weeks gestation. *Am J Perinatol* 1997;14:449-56
- Medical Devices Agency. *Report of the TINA committee.* London: Medical Devices Agency, 1995
- Leslie AJ, Stephenson TJ. Audit of neonatal intensive care transport—closing the loop. *Acta Paediatr* 1997;86:1253-6
- Davis PJ, Manktelow B, Bohin S, Field D. Paediatric trainees and the transportation of critically ill neonates: experience, training and confidence. *Acta Paediatr* 2001;90:1068-72
- Barry P, Leslie A (eds). *Paediatric and neonatal critical care transport.* London: BMJ Publishing Group, 2003

6 Respiratory complications of preterm birth

Jenny Fraser, Moira Walls, William McGuire

Respiratory complications of preterm birth are an important cause of infant mortality and morbidity. This article looks at how advances in perinatal care have improved outcomes for preterm infants with respiratory distress syndrome and chronic lung disease.

Respiratory distress syndrome

Respiratory distress syndrome of prematurity is a major cause of morbidity and mortality in preterm infants. Primarily, respiratory distress syndrome is caused by deficiency of pulmonary surfactant. Surfactant is a complex mixture of phospholipids and proteins that reduces alveolar surface tension and maintains alveolar stability. As most alveolar surfactant is produced after about 30-32 weeks' gestation, preterm infants born before then will probably develop respiratory distress syndrome. In addition to short gestation, several other clinical risk factors have been identified.

Preterm infants with respiratory distress syndrome present immediately or soon after birth with worsening respiratory distress. The presenting features include tachypnoea (respiratory rate >60 breaths per minute); intercostal, subcostal, and sternal recession; expiratory grunting; cyanosis; and diminished breath sounds.

If untreated, infants may become fatigued, apnoeic, and hypoxic. They may progress to respiratory failure and will need assisted ventilation. High airway pressures may be required to ventilate the stiff, non-compliant lungs, thereby increasing the risk of acute respiratory complications, such as pneumothorax, pneumomediastinum, and pulmonary interstitial emphysema.

Over the past 20-30 years, two major advances in perinatal management—the use of antenatal corticosteroids and exogenous surfactant replacement—have greatly improved clinical outcomes for preterm infants with respiratory distress syndrome.

Antenatal corticosteroids

Corticosteroids that cross the placenta (dexamethasone or betamethasone) given to women at risk of preterm delivery accelerate fetal surfactant production and lung maturation. The beneficial effects for preterm infants, including a 40% reduced risk of mortality, respiratory distress syndrome, and intraventricular haemorrhage were defined in randomised controlled trials throughout the 1970s and 1980s. The meta-analysis of these trials is a landmark in evidence based perinatal care. Despite the accumulation of such convincing evidence, it is only in the past decade that antenatal corticosteroids have become widely used in clinical practice.

The effect of antenatal corticosteroids lasts about a week. A Cochrane systematic review concludes that there is insufficient evidence on the benefits and risks (possible adverse effects on the developing fetal brain) to recommend repeated doses of antenatal corticosteroids for women who have not delivered in one week of the initial course. This clinical uncertainty may be resolved when the results of further trials are available.

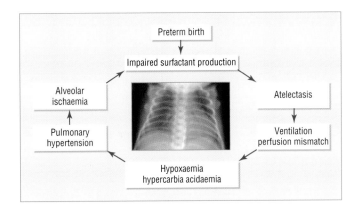

Pathogenesis of respiratory distress syndrome is a "vicious cycle"

Risk factors for respiratory distress syndrome

- Male sex
- White ethnic group
- Maternal diabetes
- Perinatal asphyxia
- Hypothermia
- Multifetal pregnancy
- Delivery by caesarean section

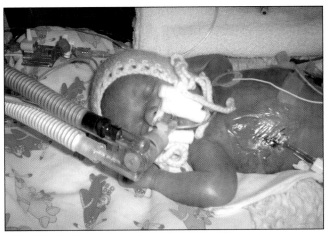

Endotracheal intubation and ventilation: intercostal drain for pneumothorax

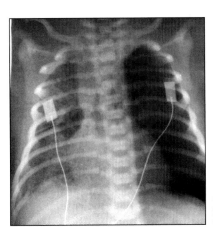

Chest x ray of left pneumothorax (undrained)

Surfactant replacement

Exogenous surfactant, given via an endotracheal tube, for the treatment or prophylaxis of respiratory distress syndrome is associated with a 40% reduction in neonatal mortality and a 30% to 65% reduction in the risk of pneumothorax. In infants at risk of developing respiratory distress syndrome, surfactant replacement is most effective when given at the time of delivery (prophylactic), rather than when symptoms develop (rescue). Treatment with repeated doses of surfactant improves survival compared with single dose treatment in infants with ongoing respiratory distress. Comparative trials have also shown that the use of natural surfactant extracts, usually porcine or bovine, is associated with a lower rate of mortality than if synthetic surfactant products are used.

Mechanical ventilation

Preterm infants with respiratory distress syndrome often require a period of assisted ventilatory support. The aim is to treat hypoxaemia and hypercarbia while minimising ventilator associated lung trauma and oxygen toxicity.

In conventional mechanical ventilation, the positive pressure ventilator delivers a given number of breaths (for a set inspiratory time at a set pressure) regardless of the baby's inspiratory effort. Ventilating preterm babies at fast rates (>40 breaths per minute) and with short inspiratory times (<0.4 seconds) reduces the risk of pneumothorax probably because the ventilator inflations are more synchronous with the infant's own respiratory cycle.

Modern ventilators can be set to trigger or to integrate with the baby's inspiratory effort (patient triggered ventilation). High frequency oscillator and jet ventilators deliver extremely rapid rates (about 600-800 breaths per minute) of very small tidal volumes. Although the results of physiological studies have indicated that these newer ventilators may have advantages over conventional mechanical ventilation, randomised controlled trials have not provided any convincing evidence of clinically important benefits in the routine management of acute respiratory distress syndrome.

The available evidence from randomised controlled trials does not support the routine use of sedation (with intravenous opiate or benzodiazepine), or of neuromuscular blocking agents in ventilated preterm infants.

Continuous positive airway pressure

The simplest and least invasive type of ventilator provides nasal continuous positive airway pressure (nCPAP). These ventilators provide a constant end distending pressure to maintain alveolar recruitment, prevent atelectasis, and improve gas exchange.

After a period of endotracheal positive pressure ventilation, nCPAP is effective in preventing failure of extubation in preterm infants. Cohort studies have also showed that early use of nCPAP in preterm infants with respiratory distress syndrome may reduce the need for endotracheal intubation for positive pressure ventilation. Randomised trials are needed to determine the relative benefits and risks of prophylactic nCPAP in preterm infants, and to establish the optimal mode and timing of nCPAP use. These trials should also explore the effect of administering exogenous surfactant in association with nCPAP. Data from animal studies, and preliminary data from a randomised controlled trial, have provided some evidence that nCPAP combined with prophylactic surfactant might further reduce the need for endotracheal intubation and positive pressure ventilation.

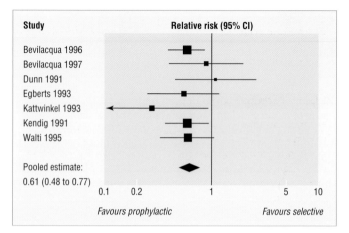

Meta-analysis of prophylactic versus selective use of surfactant to prevent mortality in preterm infants. Adapted from Soll et al. *Cochrane Database Syst Rev* 2003;(4):CD000510

Indications for mechanical ventilation in preterm infants with respiratory distress syndrome

- Hypoxaemia (paO$_2$ < 50 mmHg)
- Hypercarbia (paCO$_2$ > 50 mmHg)
- Acidosis (pH < 7.25)
- Cardiorespiratory collapse
- Persistent apnoea or bradycardia

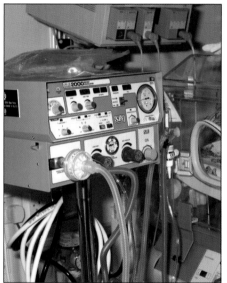

Conventional mechanical ventilators are usually set to deliver a given number of breaths for a set inspiratory time at a set pressure

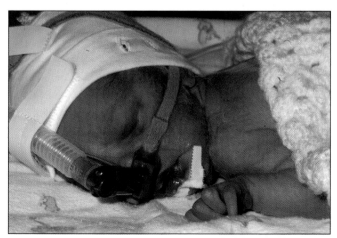

Nasal continuous positive airway pressure can be delivered via sealed nasal prongs or a nasal mask without the need for endotracheal intubation

Nitric oxide

The available evidence from randomised controlled trials does not support the use of inhaled nitric oxide in preterm infants with hypoxic respiratory failure.

Apnoea of prematurity

Very preterm infants have an immature central respiratory drive and are susceptible to episodes of apnoea that may result in a need for further mechanical ventilation. Methylxanthines (including caffeine) are effective in preventing and treating apnoea of prematurity, but their effect on longer term outcomes (including neurodevelopment) are not yet known.

Chronic lung disease

The most important long term complication of respiratory

Risk factors for chronic lung disease

- Short gestation
- Small for gestational age
- Severity of respiratory distress syndrome
- Duration of mechanical ventilation
- Duration of oxygen administration
- Patent ductus arteriosus
- Maternal chorioamnionitis
- Postnatal sepsis

---

distress syndrome is chronic lung disease of prematurity, which is usually defined as a need for ventilatory support or supplemental oxygen at 36 weeks after conception. The risk of chronic lung disease is related to the degree of prematurity and severity of the initial lung disease and to the duration of mechanical ventilation and oxygen administration. Despite the use of antenatal corticosteroids and surfactant replacement, the incidence of chronic lung disease has continued to rise over the past decade, possibly because of the increased survival of extremely preterm infants.

Postnatal steroids for chronic lung disease

Because inflammation (secondary to infection and ventilator induced lung damage) may be an important part of the disease process, corticosteroids have been used for prophylaxis and treatment of evolving or established chronic lung disease. Although systemic corticosteroids (dexamethasone or betamethasone) may have short term benefits such as earlier endotracheal extubation, there are also short term complications. These complications include hypertension, hyperglycaemia, gastrointestinal bleeding, hypertrophic cardiomyopathy, infection, and adrenal suppression. Additionally, recent studies in animal models and meta-analyses of clinical trials have highlighted concerns about long term complications, including poor brain growth and adverse developmental and neuromotor outcomes, including cerebral palsy.

The risk of adverse longer term outcomes seems to be greatest when corticosteroids are prescribed in the first few days after birth (prophylaxis). Data with regard to long term neurodevelopment when infants receive therapeutic corticosteroids after the first week of life are more reassuring. Until further evidence has been obtained, corticosteroids should be prescribed in exceptional circumstances only and after discussion of the possible risks with the infant's parents.

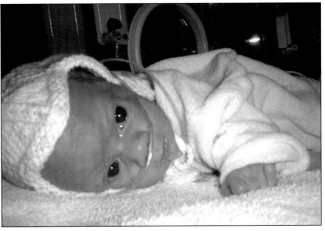

Infant with chronic lung disease (nasal prongs for oxygen)—chronic lung disease develops in about one quarter of preterm infants who receive positive pressure ventilation for respiratory distress syndrome

---

Outside the context of a randomised, controlled trial the use of corticosteroids should be limited to exceptional clinical circumstances—for example, an infant on maximal ventilatory and oxygen support. In those circumstances, parents should be fully informed about the known short and long term risks and agree to treatment—American Academy of Pediatrics Committee on Fetus and Newborn. *Pediatrics* **2002;109:330-8**

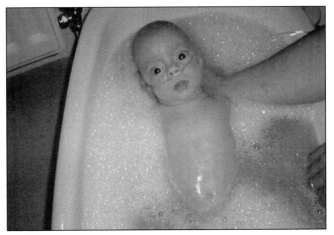

Planning for home oxygen treatment needs to be carefully coordinated and should include a programme of education and training for all members of family who will be caring for the baby

---

Preparation for home oxygen treatment

- Parental training—how to monitor respiratory status, when to provide extra oxygen, when and where to get help, cardiorespiratory resuscitation
- Family support—usually from community nurse
- Risk assessment of the home environment
- Insurance of car and house
- Notify fire and ambulance services
- Financial help—disability parking permits, disability living allowances

Inhaled corticosteroids

Little evidence exists to support the use of nebulised corticosteroids for preterm infants with evolving or established respiratory distress syndrome, although their use in ventilated infants with chronic lung disease may allow earlier extubation.

Diuretics for chronic lung disease

Diuretics are often used to treat infants with chronic lung disease because they reduce pulmonary oedema, decrease oxygen requirements, and improve lung compliance. Diuretics, however, also cause electrolyte disturbances, bone loss, and nephrocalcinosis. Furthermore, there is little evidence that the use of diuretics has any long term clinically important benefits in preterm infants with chronic lung disease.

Home oxygen treatment

Infants with chronic lung disease, who remain dependent on supplemental oxygen to maintain appropriate oxygen saturation, but who are otherwise ready for discharge home, may be suitable for home oxygen treatment. Home oxygen treatment programmes are delivered by a multidisciplinary team that includes the family plus key staff from hospital, primary care, and pharmacy services.

After discharge home, infants with chronic lung disease have a higher risk of rehospitalisation with respiratory illness than infants of the same gestational age who do not have chronic lung disease. For example, one in eight infants with chronic lung disease requires readmission to hospital for respiratory syncitial virus bronchiolitis. Immunoprophylaxis with anti-respiratory syncitial virus antibodies may reduce hospital readmission rates. It is expensive, however, and has not been shown to be effective in reducing mortality or major morbidity, such as the need for mechanical ventilation. Parents can be reassured that infants with chronic lung disease have few clinically important respiratory problems in later childhood.

Conclusion

Advances in perinatal care, particularly the use of mechanical ventilation, antenatal steroids, and exogenous surfactant replacement have improved outcomes for preterm infants. The incidence of chronic lung disease has not decreased, however, and further research is needed to define safe and effective ways to prevent and treat this condition. These efforts should continue in parallel with the development and evaluation of family centred treatments for chronic lung disease, such as home oxygen treatment programmes.

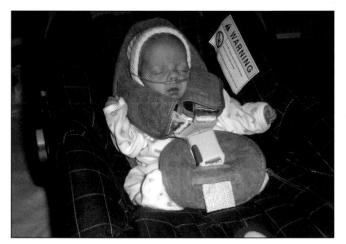

Home oxygen treatment allows earlier hospital discharge but parents are committed to the programme for at least several months while the supplemental oxygen is gradually reduced

Further reading

- Crowley P. Prophylactic corticosteroids for preterm birth. *Cochrane Database Syst Rev* 2003;(4):CD000065
- Soll RF, Morley CJ. Prophylactic versus selective use of surfactant in preventing morbidity and mortality in preterm infants. *Cochrane Database Syst Rev* 2003;(4):CD000510
- Greenough A, Milner AD, Dimitriou G. Synchronized mechanical ventilation for respiratory support in newborn infants. *Cochrane Database Syst Rev* 2003;(4):CD000456
- Henderson-Smart DJ, Bhuta T, Cools F, Offringa M. Elective high frequency oscillatory ventilation versus conventional ventilation for acute pulmonary dysfunction in preterm infants. *Cochrane Database Syst Rev* 2003;(4):CD000104
- Halliday HL, Ehrenkranz RA. Moderately early postnatal (7-14 days) corticosteroids for preventing chronic lung disease in preterm infants. *Cochrane Database Syst Rev* 2003;(1):CD001144
- Brion LP, Primhak RA, Ambrosio-Perez I. Diuretics acting on the distal renal tubule for preterm infants with (or developing) chronic lung disease. *Cochrane Database Syst Rev* 2003;(4):CD001817
- Wang EEL, Tang NK. Immunoglobulin for preventing respiratory syncytial virus infection. *Cochrane Database Syst Rev* 2003;(4):CD001725

7 Care in the early newborn period

William McGuire, Peter McEwan, Peter W Fowlie

The first week after birth is a time of major metabolic and physiological adaptation for newborn infants. Preterm infants have to cope with additional stresses because most of their organ systems are immature or because of associated illnesses, such as congenital infection. Very preterm infants (< 32 weeks' gestation) or ill infants often need intensive monitoring and support during this critical period of postnatal adaptation.

Temperature control and fluid balance

Preterm infants are susceptible to heat and fluid loss, especially immediately after delivery and in the first few days after birth. Hypothermia is associated with increased morbidity and mortality. Trials in the 1950s showed that reducing heat loss improves survival for preterm and low birthweight infants. Measures to prevent cold stress should start immediately after delivery—for example, resuscitating newborns under radiant heaters, drying them, and wrapping them in warmed towels straight away. A randomised controlled trial showed that wrapping the infant in polyethylene immediately (without drying) is at least as effective in reducing evaporative heat loss in extremely preterm infants (< 28 weeks' gestation).

Maintaining the neutral thermal environment

After admission to the neonatal unit unnecessary oxygen and energy consumption must be minimised. Several options are available for nursing preterm infants in a neutral thermal environment. Bigger and more mature infants (weighing > 1800 g) can usually maintain their body temperatures in open cots with clothing (including a hat), covers, and possibly a heated mattress. Smaller and less mature infants, particularly very preterm infants, are usually cared for in air heated perspex incubators or in open cots, where they are placed under clear polyethylene blankets and there are overhead radiant heaters. The air temperature of the incubator or the power of the overhead heater can be set to respond to changes in the temperature of the infant's abdominal wall to try to maintain the infant's temperature at 36.5°C to 37°C.

Closed incubators allow adjustment of the ambient humidity, and this further reduces heat and fluid evaporation. Consequently, incubator care is associated with less insensible water loss, and lower fluid requirements, than nursing infants in open cots under radiant heaters. Both closed incubator and open cot care have other potential advantages. Environmental noise and light can be reduced with incubator care and this may improve sleep patterns. Open cots, however, allow easy access for carers. Additionally, parents might find it easier to bond with their babies if they are nursed in an open cot rather than in a closed incubator. At present there are insufficient data to determine whether open cots or incubators confer more beneficial effects on important clinical outcomes.

Preterm infants have higher fluid requirements than term infants, especially in the first week after birth, mainly because they lose more fluid through the skin and through breathing. As fluid input for preterm infants must take into account these variable losses, prescriptions are usually tailored to individual infants. Additionally, preterm infants have immature renal tubular function in the first few days after birth. This is associated with an inadequate capacity to excrete sodium and so preterm

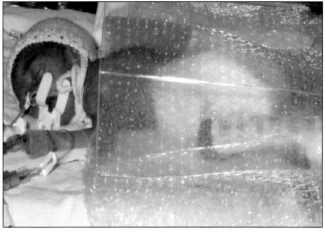

Covering the preterm infant with a polythene blanket reduces heat and fluid loss

Average fluid and electrolyte requirements in early neonatal period

Days after birth	Fluid (ml/kg/day)	Sodium (mmol/kg/day)	Potassium (mmol/kg/day)
1	60	0	0
2	90	0	0
3	120	2-3	1-2
4	120-50	3-5	1-2
5 onwards	150 +	3-5 +	1-2

Heat and fluid loss

Preterm infants are susceptible to heat and fluid loss because:
- High surface area to volume ratio
- Thin non-keratinised skin
- Lack of insulating subcutaneous fat
- Lack of thermogenic brown fat
- Inability to shiver

Potential adverse consequences of hypothermia

- High oxygen consumption can lead to hypoxia
- High use of glucose can lead to hypoglycaemia
- High energy expenditure can cause reduced rate of growth
- Low surfactant production can cause respiratory distress
- Vasoconstriction may cause poor perfusion or metabolic acidosis
- Delayed adjustment from fetal to newborn circulation

The neutral thermal environment is the ambient temperature at which oxygen consumption and energy expenditure is at the minimum to sustain vital activities

infants have a lower sodium requirement than term infants. Fluid and electrolyte balance must be monitored frequently to avoid dehydration or excessive fluid input.

Metabolic homeostasis

Hypoglycaemia is common in preterm infants, with risk inversely related to gestational age. Very preterm infants must maintain high energy output to overcome thermal stress and to support respiratory efforts. Growth restricted preterm infants are at great risk of hypoglycaemia because they have limited fat and glycogen reserves at the time of delivery.

The level or duration of hypoglycaemia that is harmful to a preterm infant's developing brain is not known. Hypoglycaemia is a potentially more serious complication for preterm infants than term infants because preterm infants have a relatively impaired ability to produce alternative brain fuels, such as ketones. Interventions, such as giving more milk or starting an intravenous glucose infusion, are necessary when the laboratory measured blood glucose level remains < 2.0 mmol/l.

Conversely, very preterm infants are also susceptible to hyperglycaemia and glycosuria, which can disturb fluid balance by inducing an osmotic diuresis. If glycosuria persists despite reducing the glucose input, insulin may be needed.

Neonatal jaundice is common in preterm infants and is treated with phototherapy at lower thresholds than in term infants because of concern that even moderate hyperbilirubinaemia may effect neurodevelopment adversely.

Haemodynamic status

Hypotension is associated with adverse outcomes, particularly intraventricular haemorrhage and periventricular leucomalacia. Hypotension and suboptimal systemic perfusion can be secondary to several problems. Management should be directed at treating the underlying cause (for example, giving volume replacement or antibiotics) and should include measures to improve systemic perfusion, such as inotrope support.

Optimal arterial blood pressure for preterm infants meets perfusion needs for vital organs. Reference ranges for blood pressure in healthy preterm infants in the first week after birth have been published. As a rule of thumb, the mean blood pressure (mmHg) should not be lower than the number of weeks of the infant's gestational age.

Although relatively easy to measure and monitor, arterial blood pressure does not correlate well with cardiac output and systemic perfusion in preterm infants. Other variables including heart rate, peripheral oxygen saturation, acid-base status, and urine output can be measured. These too are relatively poor measures of organ perfusion. Doppler ultrasonography assessments of systemic perfusion might be more useful for determining when to intervene and which intervention is most appropriate. Currently, these techniques are not widely available.

Patent ductus arteriosus

In the first few days after birth, patency of the ductus arteriosus is a major cause of hypotension and poor perfusion. Over one quarter of very preterm infants develop a clinically important patent ductus arteriosus. The risk of this is greatest in infants with severe respiratory distress syndrome. The clinical consequences are related to shunting of blood through the patent ductus from the aorta to the pulmonary arterial circulation. This "left to right" shunt alters the blood flow distribution to vital organs. Increased pulmonary blood flow can damage the preterm lungs. Preterm infants with a patent

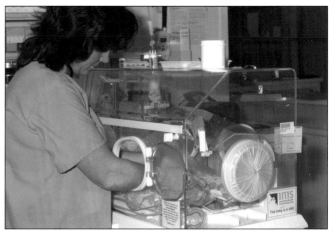

Nursing preterm infants in incubators allows the neutral thermal envrionment, noise, and light to be controlled effectively. Ports allow access to the infant

---

Risk factors for increased insensible fluid loss

- Short gestation
- High ambient temperature
- Radiant heater
- Phototherapy lamp
- Low ambient humidity

Variables that should be monitored in the very preterm infant

- Temperature: core and peripheral
- Heart rate
- Respiratory rate
- Peripheral oxygen saturation
- Blood pressure
- Urine output
- Partial pressure of oxygen and carbon dioxide
- Acid-base status
- Electrolyte balance
- Weight gain or loss

Risk factors for hypotension and poor perfusion

- Short gestational age
- Lack of antenatal steroids
- Positive pressure ventilation
- Patent ductus arteriosus
- Perinatal asphyxia
- Systemic infection

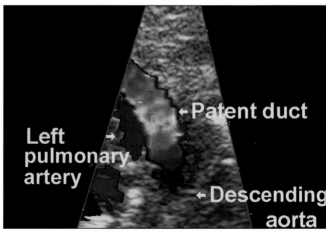

Doppler colour flow of patent ductus arteriosus with left to right shunt that can change blood flow distribution to organs. Courtesy of Drs N Evans and G Malcolm, Royal Prince Alfred Hospital, Sydney

ductus arteriosus are at higher risk of more severe and prolonged respiratory distress syndrome, chronic lung disease, intraventricular haemorrhage, and death than similar infants whose ductuses have closed.

The patent ductus arteriosus may be closed surgically, with transthoracic ligation, or pharmacologically, with prostaglandin synthase inhibitors, such as indometacin or ibuprofen. Current data on overall benefits and harms are insufficient to determine if surgical or medical treatment is the better initial treatment for symptomatic patent ductus arteriosus in preterm infants. In most centres, surgical ligation is reserved for instances where the ductus remains open despite pharmacological treatment. However, retrospective studies show that surgical ligation may be a better firstline treatment in extremely preterm infants, particularly if the ductus is large. Further randomised controlled trials are needed to clarify these issues.

Prophylaxis with indometacin

Prophylactic use of indometacin in very low birthweight infants confers short term benefits, including a fall in the incidence of symptomatic patent ductus arteriosus, a reduced need for surgical ligation, and a reduced incidence of intraventricular haemorrhage. Prophylactic indometacin does not, however, improve survival or longer term neurodevelopmental outcomes. The decision to use prophylactic indometacin will depend on the values that parents and carers attach to the short term benefits. In neonatal units without ready access to cardiac surgical services, a reduction in the need for surgical ligation may be considered a greater benefit than in units with these services.

Anaemia of prematurity

Anaemia is common in very preterm infants. Evidence exists that delaying umbilical cord clamping until 30-60 seconds after birth facilitates fetoplacental transfusion and reduces the need for blood transfusions in the early neonatal period. Further large trials are needed to clarify whether this practice improves important outcomes, such as longer term neurodevelopment for very preterm infants. Postnatally, repeated blood sampling is a major cause of anaemia of prematurity. Very preterm infants can lose 10-25% of their blood volume each week through blood sampling. Although transfusion with packed cells can replace these losses, uncertainty exists over the most appropriate indications for replacement transfusion. Given the potential complications, blood transfusions should be limited to the minimum needed to maintain optimal oxygen delivery to vital organs. Recombinant erythropoietin is an alternative to blood transfusion. Little evidence exists, however, to show that its use reduces the number of blood transfusions needed in extremely preterm infants—the population at greatest risk of anaemia of prematurity.

Conclusion

As well as respiratory and nutritional support, optimal care for preterm infants in the early neonatal period demands attention to several key inter-related issues, including temperature control, fluid and electrolyte balance, glucose homeostasis, and haemodynamic status. Maintaining metabolic and physiological stability at this time may have an important impact on survival and neurodevelopmental outcomes.

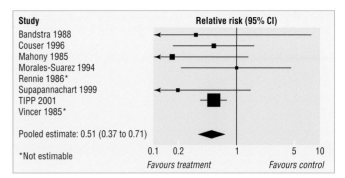

Meta-analysis of need for surgical ductus ligation in trials of prophylactic indometacin in very low birthweight infants. Adapted from Fowlie PW et al. *Cochrane Database Syst Rev* 2003;(4):CD000174

Analgesia—evidence from randomised controlled trials exists that glucose or sucrose solutions given orally reduces pain responses (particularly the duration of crying) for preterm infants undergoing procedures such as venepuncture

---

Aetiology of anaemia of prematurity
- Frequent blood sampling
- Low reticulocyte levels
- Low levels of endogenous erythropoietin
- Poor response to endogenous erythropoietin
- Shortened life span of neonatal erythrocytes

Measures to reduce the risk of infection associated with transfusion
- Screen donors for transmissible viruses
- Limit exposure to multiple donors—multiple paediatric packs from single adult donor
- Use cytomegalovirus antibody negative blood
- Irradiate transfusion packs
- Use leucocyte depletion filters (removes cytomegalovirus)

Further reading
- Flenady VJ, Woodgate PG. Radiant warmers versus incubators for regulating body temperature in newborn infants. *Cochrane Database Syst Rev.* 2003;(4):CD000435
- Cornblath M, Hawdon JM, Williams AF, Aynsley-Green A, Ward-Platt MP, Schwartz R, et al. Controversies regarding definition of neonatal hypoglycemia: suggested operational thresholds. *Pediatrics* 2000;105:1141-5
- Malviya M, Ohlsson A, Shah S. Surgical versus medical treatment with cyclo-oxygenase inhibitors for symptomatic patent ductus arteriosus in preterm infants *Cochrane Database Syst Rev.* 2003;(3):CD003951
- Fowlie PW, Davis PG. Prophylactic intravenous indomethacin for preventing mortality and morbidity in preterm infants. *Cochrane Database Syst Rev.* 2003;(4):CD000174
- Rabe H, Reynolds G, Diaz-Rossello J. Early versus delayed umbilical cord clamping in preterm infants. *Cochrane Database Syst Rev.* 2003;(3):CD003248
- Evans NJ, Malcolm G. Practical echocardiography for the neonatologist (CD Rom) (search via www.cs.nsw.gov.au/rpa/neonatal/)
- Stevens B, Yamada J, Ohlsson A. Sucrose for analgesia in newborn infants undergoing painful procedures. *Cochrane Database Syst Rev.* 2004;(3):CD001069

8 Feeding the preterm infant

William McGuire, Ginny Henderson, Peter W Fowlie

Providing appropriate nutrition for growth and development is a cornerstone of the care of preterm infants. Early postnatal nutrition during this critical period of brain growth may have a substantial impact on clinically important outcomes, including long term neurodevelopment.

Preterm infants, especially those who have been growth restricted in utero, have fewer nutrient reserves at birth than term infants. Additionally, preterm infants are subject to physiological and metabolic stresses that can affect their nutritional needs, such as respiratory distress or infection. An international consensus group has recommended nutritional requirements for preterm infants. These recommendations are based on data from intrauterine growth and nutrient balance studies and assume that the optimal rate of postnatal growth for preterm infants should be similar to that of normal fetuses of the same postconception age. In practice, however, these target levels of nutrient input are not always achieved and this may result in important nutritional deficits.

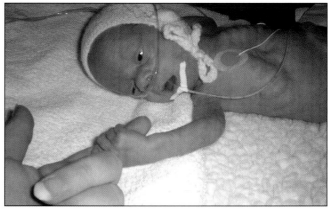
Infants with intrauterine growth restriction lack subcutaneous fat and other nutrient stores

Nutritional requirements for preterm infants*

- Energy—110-20 kcal/kg/day
- Protein—3-3.8 g/kg/day
- Fat—4.5-6.8 g/kg/day
- Calcium—120-230 mg/kg/day
- Phosphorus—60-140 mg/kg/day

*International consensus group recommendations

Enteral feeding

Well infants of gestational age > 34 weeks are usually able to coordinate sucking, swallowing, and breathing, and so establish breast or bottle feeding. In less mature infants, oral feeding may not be safe or possible because of neurological immaturity or respiratory compromise. In these infants milk can be given as a continuous infusion or as an intermittent bolus through a fine feeding catheter passed via the nose or the mouth to the stomach.

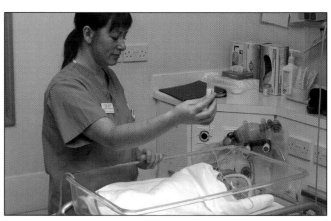
Infants can be fed using a gastric tube if they are unable to breast or bottle feed

Necrotising enterocolitis

A major concern with the introduction of enteral feeds (especially to very preterm, growth restricted, or sick infants) is that the additional physiological strain on the immature gastrointestinal tract may predispose to the development of necrotising enterocolitis. The risk of necrotising enterocolitis is inversely related to gestational age and birth weight. The incidence is 5-10% in very low birth weight infants. The mortality rate is reported consistently as greater than 20%. Long term morbidity may include substantial neurodevelopmental problems, the consequence of undernutrition and associated infection during a vulnerable period of growth and development.

Most preterm infants who develop necrotising enterocolitis have received enteral feeds. At present, however, limited evidence exists that the way that we feed infants who are at risk affects the incidence of necrotising enterocolitis. Large randomised controlled trials are needed to determine whether strategies, such as delaying the introduction of milk feeds or delivering only minimal enteral nutrition, influence clinically

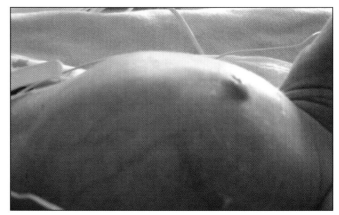
Preterm infant with necrotising enterocolitis—a syndrome of acute intestinal necrosis of unknown aetiology

Presenting clinical features of necrotising enterocolitis

- Abdominal distension
- Abdominal tenderness or rigidity
- Lethargy, hypotonia, or apnoea
- Hepatic portal gas on abdominal x ray
- Intramural gas (pneumatosis intestinalis) on abdominal x ray
- Intestinal perforation
- Blood or mucosa in stool

important outcomes for preterm infants. Apart from assessing the impact of feeding strategies on short term outcomes, such as growth, and the risk of necrotising enterocolitis, trials should also determine how various enteral feeding strategies affect mortality and long term neurodevelopment.

Which milk?

Human breast milk is the recommended form of enteral nutrition for preterm infants. The milk could be from the infant's mother or expressed milk from donor mothers, who are usually mothers who have delivered term infants. The nutrient content of expressed breast milk varies depending on the stage of lactation at which it is collected. Milk expressed from a donor's lactating breast has a higher calorie and protein content than that collected from the opposite breast (drip breast milk).

Human breast milk, particularly donated drip breast milk, may not consistently provide all of the nutrient requirements of preterm infants. Multinutrient fortifiers are available to add to human milk to achieve these targets. Fortification of human milk with calcium and phosphate may improve bone mineral content. Protein and energy supplementation of human milk increases the rate of weight gain and head growth, at least in the short term. Long term follow up studies are needed to determine if nutrient fortification of human milk improves neurodevelopmental outcomes for preterm infants.

Human breast milk has non-nutrient advantages for preterm infants, primarily through the delivery of immunoprotective and growth factors to the immature gut mucosa. Some evidence exists that preterm infants who receive human breast milk rather than formula milk have a lower incidence of feed intolerance and gastrointestinal upset, and a lower incidence of necrotising enterocolitis.

Supporting mothers to express breast milk

Mothers may be very anxious after preterm delivery, especially if their infant needs intensive care. Although feeding might not be seen as an immediate concern, mothers should be aware that providing breast milk is one of the most important parts of their infant's care. In developing countries, supporting mothers to provide expressed breast milk may be the most important intervention available for preterm infants. Feeding with expressed human milk reduces the risk of serious infection, which is a major cause of neonatal morbidity and mortality in preterm infants in developing countries.

Various initiatives may help mothers who are expressing breast milk:
- Early discussion of breast feeding
- Written information
- Frequent expression
- Simultaneous expression of both breasts
- Breast massage
- Use of electric pump
- Skin to skin contact
- Sucking from as early as 32 weeks after conception
- Cup feeding
- Continued support and education.

The initiation of skin to skin contact between mother and infant (although not always possible for lengthy periods of time with extremely preterm infants) can help with bonding, milk production, and the subsequent establishment of breast feeding. Milk can be delivered via a gastric tube or by cup feeding while the infant is learning to suck at the breast. Bottle feeding should be avoided as it may interfere with the establishment of breast feeding.

Minimal enteral nutrition—main points
- Also called trophic feeding, gut priming, hypocaloric feeding
- Feeds nutritionally insignificant volumes of enteral milk (0.5-1.0 ml/hour)
- Aims to stimulate postnatal development of gastrointestinal system
- Used in parallel with total parenteral nutrition
- Enteral feeds' volume increases after prespecified interval, typically 7-14 days

---

Typical nutritional contents of human expressed breast milk (per 100 ml)*

	Milk expressed from lactating breast	Drip milk expressed from opposite breast
Energy (kcal)	73	54
Protein (g)	2.7	1.3
Fat (g)	3.0	2.2
Calcium (mg)	29	28
Phosphate (mg)	15	14

*Data from Rennie J, Robertson NRC. *A manual of neonatal intensive care*, 4th ed, London: Arnold, 2002

Osteomalacia (rickets) of prematurity is generally caused by mineral, particularly phosphate, deficiency. Extremely preterm infants are at greatest risk—enteral or parenteral mineral supplementation increases bone mineral content and reduces the incidence of rickets

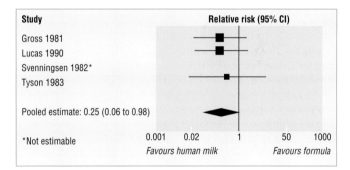

Relative risk of confirmed necrotising enterocolitis with human milk versus formula. Adapted from McGuire W, Anthony MY. *Arch Dis Child* 2003;88:11-14

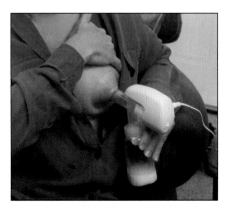

Human breast milk can be expressed from the infant's mother or from a donor mother

Donor milk banking

Use of donor milk for preterm infants has declined over the past 20 years. This fall is caused by concerns about the nutritional adequacy of donor breast milk, the resources needed to pasteurise and store donated milk, and the cost and feasibility of screening donors for transmissible infections, such as the human immunodeficiency virus. In several countries, efforts have been made to re-establish donor milk banks that were closed in the 1980s. Economic studies show that the costs of this service may be balanced by the potential health gains associated with feeding with human milk—for example, a shorter stay in hospital.

Formula milks

Despite optimal maternal support, expressed breast milk may not always be available. As an alternative, preterm infants may be fed with a variety of artificial formula milks, mainly modified cow's milk. Broadly, these may be "term" formulae (based on the composition of mature breast milk), or calorie, protein, and mineral enriched "preterm" formulae (tailored to support intrauterine nutrient accretion rates). Some evidence exists that feeding very preterm infants with preterm formula milk increases the rate of weight gain and head growth, at least in the short term, and improves some neurodevelopmental outcomes. No evidence exists that feeding preterm infants with formula milk supplemented with long chain polyunsaturated fatty acids is beneficial.

Parenteral nutrition

Very preterm infants, who often have relatively delayed gastric emptying and intestinal peristalsis, may be slow to tolerate the introduction of gastric tube feeds. These infants may need intravenous nutrition while enteral nutrition is being established or when enteral nutrition is not possible—for example, because of respiratory instability, feed intolerance, or serious gastrointestinal disease.

Total parenteral nutrition consists of a glucose and amino acid solution with electrolytes, minerals, and vitamins, plus fat as the principal non-protein energy source. The solutions are usually prepared in a specialist pharmacy to minimise the risk of microbial contamination. Bloodstream infection is the most common important complication of parenteral nutrition use. Delivery of the solution via a central venous catheter rather than a peripheral catheter is not associated with a higher risk of infection. Extravasation injury is a major concern when parenteral nutrition is given via a peripheral cannula. Subcutaneous infiltration of a hypertonic and irritant solution can cause local skin ulceration, secondary infection, and scarring.

Nutrition after hospital discharge

Most preterm infants, and especially very preterm infants, have an accumulated nutritional deficit when they are discharged from hospital. Iron and vitamin supplementation is necessary until infants are at least six months old, especially if they are fed on breast milk only. Protein and energy enriched formula milk may improve catch-up growth, at least in the short term. This may be of particular importance for infants with additional metabolic requirements, such as those caused by chronic lung disease. Further research is needed to determine if breast milk should be fortified after the infant is discharged.

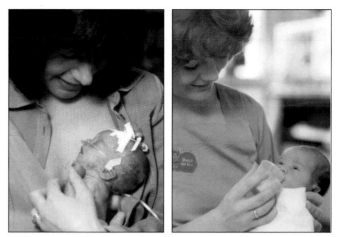

Skin to skin care may promote bonding and milk production (left). The infant can be cup fed (right) until breast feeding is established

Typical content of nutrient enriched preterm formula milk compared with standard term formula (per 100 ml)*

	Preterm formula	Term formula
Energy (kcal)	80	67
Protein (g)	2.0	1.4
Fat (g)	4.5	3.6
Calcium (mg)	77-110	39-66
Phosphate (mg)	33-63	27-42

*Data from Rennie J, Robertson NRC. *A manual of neonatal intensive care*, 4th ed, London: Arnold, 2002

Complications of total parenteral nutrition

Catheter related complications
- Bacteraemia (staphylococcal)
- Invasive fungal infection
- Thrombosis
- Extravasation injuries
- Cardiac tamponade

Metabolic complications
- Cholestatic jaundice
- Hyperglycaemia or glycosuria
- Vitamin deficiencies or excesses
- Hyperammonaemia

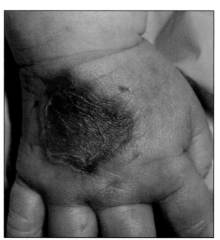

Extravasation injury may occur when a peripheral cannula is used to deliver the parenteral nutrition solution

Conclusion

The nutritional management of preterm infants may have a major impact on growth and development. Various feeding strategies are available, including the use of expressed maternal milk, donor human milk, breast milk fortifiers, adapted formula milks, and total parenteral nutrition. A lack of robust evidence exists to guide practice for many of these interventions. Large, pragmatic randomised controlled trials are needed to assess the effects of a number of these feeding strategies on clinically important outcomes for preterm infants.

The photographs showing a woman expressing breast milk, skin to skin contact, and cup feeding are courtesy of the Health Promotion Agency for Northern Ireland.

Further reading

- Ainsworth SB, Clerihew L, McGuire W. Percutaneous central venous catheters versus peripheral cannulae for delivery of parenteral nutrition in neonates. *Cochrane Database Syst Rev* 2004;(2):CD004219
- Kennedy KA, Tyson JE, Chamnanvanakij S. Rapid versus slow rate of advancement of feedings for promoting growth and preventing necrotizing enterocolitis in parenterally fed low-birth-weight infant. *Cochrane Database Syst Rev* 2003;(4):CD001241
- Kennedy KA, Tyson JE, Chamnanvanikij S. Early versus delayed initiation of progressive enteral feedings for parenterally fed low birth weight or preterm infants. *Cochrane Database Syst Rev* 2003;(4):CD001970
- Tyson JE, Kennedy KA. Minimal enteral nutrition for promoting feeding tolerance and preventing morbidity in parenterally fed infants. *Cochrane Database Syst Rev* 2004;(2):CD000504
- Morley R, Lucas A. Randomized diet in the neonatal period and growth performance until 7.5-8 years of age in preterm children. *Am J Clin Nutr* 2000;71:822-8
- Lucas A, Morley R, Cole TJ. Randomised trial of early diet in preterm babies and later intelligence quotient. *BMJ* 1998;317:1481-7
- Cooke RJ, Embleton ND. Feeding issues in preterm infants. *Arch Dis Child* 2000;83:215-8
- McGuire W, Anthony MY. Formula milk versus term human milk for feeding preterm or low birth weight infants. *Cochrane Database Syst Rev* 2003;(4):CD002972

9 Infection in the preterm infant

William McGuire, Linda Clerihew, Peter W Fowlie

Systemic infection in preterm infants has two categories with distinct aetiologies and outcomes.

Early onset infection—acquired in the intrapartum period and presenting in the first 48-72 hours after birth.

Late onset infection—usually acquired in hospital and clinically evident more than 72 hours after birth (usually after the first week of life).

Early onset infection

Incidence

Early onset systemic infection includes bacteraemia, pneumonia, meningitis, and urinary tract infection. Although rare, early onset infection is a serious complication of preterm birth. In North America the incidence of bacteraemia proved by culture in very low birthweight (< 1500 g) infants is 1.5% of live births. The principal pathogens responsible are Group B streptococci and *Escherichia coli*. Congenital listeriosis (caused by spread of *Listeria monocytogenes* across the placenta after the mother has eaten infected food) is rare in North America and the United Kingdom but more common in some areas in Europe.

In many developed countries the incidence of Group B streptococcal infection has fallen in the past decade, perhaps because of the greater use of intrapartum antibiotic treatment for women with specific risk factors. During this period, however, there has been a rise in the incidence of infection with Gram negative coliforms. Microbiological surveillance should be continued to identify changes in the epidemiology of early onset infection, particularly antibiotic resistance.

Presentation and treatment

Most infants with early onset systemic infection will present with signs of sepsis, such as respiratory distress or fever, in the first 12 hours after birth. Presentation can be delayed, and microbiological diagnosis may be difficult, especially if the mother has received intrapartum antibiotics. As it is difficult to rule out systemic infection in the symptomatic preterm neonate, empirical antibiotic treatment is given to all preterm infants with signs consistent with sepsis. Empirical antibiotic treatment is often indicated for preterm infants who seem well but who have specific risk factors for systemic infection, such as prolonged rupture of amniotic membranes.

Intravenous penicillin plus an aminoglycoside, such as gentamicin, is the commonly used firstline antibiotic regimen for suspected early onset systemic infection. In an asymptomatic infant, if blood, urine, or cerebrospinal fluid examination and cultures do not confirm infection, antibiotics are often stopped after 48 hours. Parenteral antibiotics are continued for up to 14 days when bacteraemia is confirmed, and for up to three weeks in infants with meningitis. If listeriosis is suspected then ampicillin is often substituted for penicillin, although both are probably equally effective. *L monocytogenes* is, however, resistant to all cephalosporins.

Mortality in very low birthweight infants with early onset systemic infection is close to 40%, three times higher than in infants of the same gestation without infection. Congenital listeriosis is associated with a mortality rate of about 50%. Early

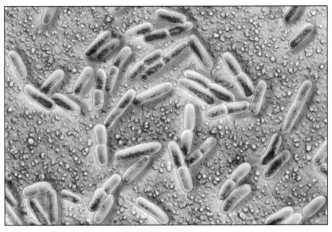

Gram negative bacilli, particularly *E coli*, are an increasingly common cause of early onset infection in very low birthweight infants

Micro-organisms causing early onset infection in very low birthweight infants*

	Rate per 1000 live born infants	
	1991-93	1998-2000
Group B streptococcus	5.9	1.7
Other Gram positive organisms	5.0	4.0
E coli	3.2	6.8
Other Gram negative organisms	5.1	2.6

* Adapted from Stoll BJ, et al. *N Engl J Med* 2002;347:240-7

Risk factors for early onset Group B streptococcal infection in preterm infants

- Group B streptococcal infection in mother's previous baby
- Group B streptococcal infection in mother's vagina or urine during pregnancy
- Mother has fever during labour
- Prolonged rupture of amniotic membranes (> 18 hours)

Presenting features of early onset systemic infection in preterm infants

- Respiratory distress
- Unstable temperature
- Floppiness
- Irritability
- Poor feeding
- Early onset jaundice
- Apnoea
- Poor perfusion
- Tachycardia
- Seizures

onset systemic infection, particularly meningitis, is also associated with a high incidence of neurodevelopmental impairment, including cerebral palsy, and visual and hearing impairment in surviving children. The appropriate use of preventive strategies, such as intrapartum antibiotic prophylaxis, and the early empirical treatment of infected infants, may help reduce the incidence and severity of such adverse outcomes.

Late onset infection

Incidence
In contrast to early onset infection, late onset infection acquired in hospital is common, occurring in about 20% of very low birthweight infants. Most infections are caused by Gram positive organisms. Coagulase negative staphylococci account for half of all late onset infections. Risk of infection is inversely related to gestational age and birth weight, and directly related to the severity of illness at birth. These risk factors reflect the need for invasive interventions such as prolonged ventilation or vascular access. Late onset systemic infection with Gram negative organisms is often associated with specific complications of preterm birth, such as urinary tract infection.

Nosocomial infection is the most common serious complication related to central venous catheters ("long lines"), which are often used to deliver parenteral nutrition to preterm infants. It is uncertain, however, whether using central venous catheters further increases the risk of infection in a population that is already at risk. The central venous catheter, or an associated thrombus, can act as a nidus for infection. The catheter may need to be removed to clear the infection.

Presentation and treatment
The clinical presentation of systemic infection, particularly with coagulase negative staphylococci, can be insidious. Diagnosis depends on the early recognition of presenting clinical and laboratory signs.

Clinical signs include:
- Increasing apnoea
- Feeding intolerance or abdominal distension
- Increased respiratory support
- Lethargy and hypotonia.

Laboratory signs include:
- Abnormal white blood cell count
- Unexplained metabolic acidosis
- Hyperglycaemia.

Good management includes the early investigation of suspected infection (a chest x ray is needed if pneumonia is suspected), and microbiological culture of blood, urine, and cerebrospinal fluid if meningitis is suspected.

Coagulase negative staphylococci are skin commensals and may contaminate samples that have been taken inappropriately. Conversely, blood samples that are of insufficient volume may give falsely reassuring negative results on culture. Blood samples for microbial culture (ideally, at least 1 ml) should be obtained from peripheral sites rather than indwelling cannulas. Urine should be obtained by suprapubic aspiration or "in out" aseptic catheterisation of the bladder.

Antibiotic treatment is usually started as soon as these investigations have been done, and stopped when appropriate cultures are confirmed as negative—usually after 48 hours. As antibiotics are often prescribed empirically for infants with suspected sepsis, their rational use is essential to limit the emergence of antibiotic resistant bacteria. The firstline treatment for suspected nosocomial sepsis in preterm infants should include an antistaphylococcal antibiotic, such as flucloxacillin, and an aminoglycoside. Flucloxacillin, however, is

---

Main organisms causing late onset systemic infection in very low birthweight infants

Gram positive organisms
- Coagulase negative staphylococci
- *Staphylococcus aureus*
- Enterococci

Gram negative organisms
- *E coli*
- *Klebsiella* spp
- *Pseudomonas* spp

Fungi
- Mainly *Candida* spp

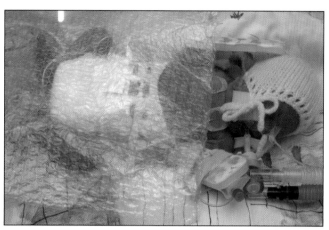

A preterm infant may need invasive interventions, such as ventilation and vascular access, which may increase the risk of infection

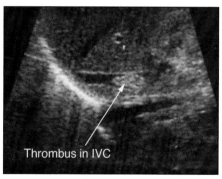

Central venous catheters, often used to deliver parenteral nutrition to preterm infants, can act as a nidus for infection. This ultrasonogram shows a long line associated (infected) thrombus in the inferior vena cava (IVC)

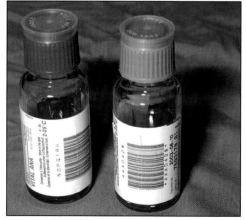

If a blood sample of insufficient volume is obtained the result may be false negative. Skin contaminants in samples that have been taken inappropriately may give false positive results

not active (at least in vitro) against coagulase negative staphylococci. Vancomycin or teicoplanin is indicated for an infant with confirmed, or strongly suspected, coagulase negative staphylococcal infection, or in infants with a poor response to firstline antibiotics.

The high mortality in preterm infants with late onset infection is mainly associated with Gram negative coliform infection, or with invasive fungal infection. Coagulase negative staphylococcal infection, although common, is associated with a more benign clinical course. Meningitis is rare and associated mortality is lower than with infection from other organisms. Inflammatory cascades associated with even "low grade" systemic infection may play a part in the pathogenesis of white matter and other brain damage that may result in neurodevelopmental impairment. Preterm infants who acquire infection in hospital have substantially prolonged hospital stays. This has important implications for resources and costs in health services

Invasive fungal infection

The clinical presentation of invasive fungal and bacterial infection is similar, and this may cause a delay in diagnosis and treatment. The diagnosis may be further delayed if the organism cannot be recovered consistently from blood, cerebrospinal fluid, or urine. A high index of suspicion and the use of additional clinical tests, including retinal examination, echocardiography, and renal ultrasonography, may be needed to confirm the suspected diagnosis. Although systemic antifungal treatment is often given before the diagnosis is confirmed, about one third of very low birthweight infants with invasive fungal infection die. The role of prophylactic antifungal treatment for preterm infants at high risk of invasive fungal infection is still unclear. Topical prophylaxis (for example, with nystatin) can reduce fungal colonisation and infection. Some evidence shows that systemic prophylaxis with fluconazole reduces the incidence of invasive fungal infection, and possibly the mortality rate in very low birthweight infants. The effect of this intervention on longer term outcomes, including neurodevelopment and the emergence of antifungal resistance, is still to be determined.

Adjunctive treatments for systemic infection

Because of the high mortality and morbidity associated with systemic infection in preterm infants, even with appropriate antibiotic treatment, adjunctive therapies that might improve outcomes have been sought. Recent attention has focused on the potential role of immunomodulatory drugs, and several large multicentre randomised controlled trials of these interventions are under way. Proposed adjuvant therapies for sepsis in preterm infants include:
- Polyclonal immunoglobulin
- Colony stimulating factors—for example, granulocyte-macrophage colony stimulating factor (GM-CSF)
- Granulocyte transfusions
- Anticytokine treatments.

Prevention of nosocomial infection

The impact of infection control practices may be affected by organisational issues (such as the layout of the neonatal intensive care unit, staffing levels, and throughput of patients) as well as training and educational factors. Continued research at all of these levels is needed if efforts to reduce the burden of infection in preterm infants are to be successful.

Some specific infection control practices, such as aseptic handling of central venous catheters and compliance with hand washing, are effective in reducing the incidence of hospital acquired infection in preterm infants.

> The overall mortality rate in preterm infants with late onset systemic infection is substantially higher than in those without infection

Risk factors for invasive fungal infection in very low birthweight infants
- Fungal colonisation
- Severe illness at birth
- Use of multiple courses of antibiotics, especially third generation cephalosporins
- Use of parenteral nutrition
- Presence of a central venous catheter
- Use of H_2 receptor antagonists

Antifungal treatments for preterm infants
- Amphotericin B
- Lipid complex amphotericin B
- 5-Fluorocytosine (flucytosine)
- Triazoles (fluconazole, itraconazole)
- Imidazoles (miconazole, ketoconazole)

> Invasive fungal infection, mainly caused by *Candida* spp, accounts for about 10% of all cases of late onset sepsis in preterm infants

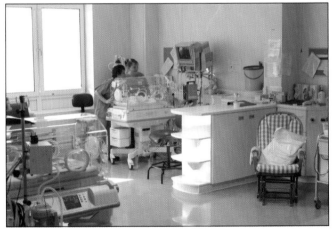

The layout and organisation of the neonatal unit may have an important effect on infection control practices

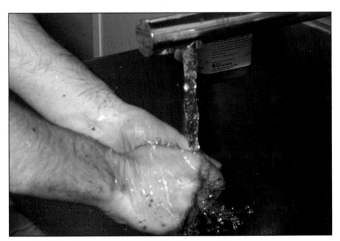

Hand washing is a cornerstone of infection control

Recent research has indicated that the routine use of alcohol solutions as hand rubs after any patient contact may achieve a greater reduction in bacterial contamination of hands than conventional washing with medicated soap. Other measures, such as routine use of gowns, hats, and masks by staff or parents, are much less effective in preventing infection. The use of prophylactic antibiotics is not substantially beneficial for very low birthweight infants, and may contribute to the emergence of antibiotic resistant bacteria in the neonatal intensive care unit.

Conclusion

Systemic infection, particularly nosocomial infection, is an important cause of morbidity and mortality in preterm infants. Infants born after very short gestations and require intensive care and undergo invasive procedures are most at risk. Clinical and laboratory diagnosis can be difficult, potentially leading to delayed treatment. New prevention and treatment strategies are needed because morbidity is high despite antimicrobial treatment.

Further reading

- Stoll BJ, Hansen N, Fanaroff AA, Wright LL, Carlo WA, Ehrenkranz RA, et al. Late-onset sepsis in very low birth weight neonates: the experience of the NICHD Neonatal Research Network. *Pediatrics* 2002;110:285-91
- Stoll BJ, Hansen N, Fanaroff AA, Wright LL, Carlo WA, Ehrenkranz RA, et al Changes in pathogens causing early-onset sepsis in very-low-birth-weight infants. *N Engl J Med* 2002;347:240-7
- Fanaroff AA, Korones SB, Wright LL, Verter J, Poland RL, Bauer O, et al. Incidence, presenting features, risk factors and significance of late onset septicaemia in very low birth weight infants. The National Institute of Child Health and Human Development Neonatal Research Network. *Pediatr Infect Dis J* 1998;17:593-8
- Saiman L, Ludington E, Pfaller M, Rangel-Fraustro S, Wilbin TR, Dawson J, et al. Risk factors for candidemia in neonatal intensive care unit patients. The National Epidemiology of Mycosis Survey Study Group. *Pediatr Infect Dis J* 2000; 19:319-24
- Adams-Chapman I, Stoll BJ. Prevention of nosocomial infections in the neonatal intensive care unit. *Curr Opin Pediatr* 2002;14:157-64

Competing interests: WMcG received a grant from Pfizer UK for a national study of fungal infection in preterm infants.

The coloured scanning electron micrograph of *Escherichia coli* bacteria is with permission of BSIP/Science Photo Library. The ultrasonogram showing long line associated (infected) thrombus in inferior vena cava is courtesy of Dr Gavin Main.

10   Supporting parents in the neonatal unit

Peter W Fowlie, Hazel McHaffie

Parents find it very stressful when their baby is admitted to the neonatal unit for any reason. Different sources of stress have been identified, and certain occasions (such as discharge from hospital or bereavement) are particularly difficult. These experiences impact on families in positive and negative ways, and people adopt a range of coping mechanisms. Staff should adopt a holistic approach to care that acknowledges the uniqueness of each family and supports them appropriately.

Sources of stress

During pregnancy, most women and their partners do not give serious consideration to the possibility of preterm delivery or illness in their newborn baby. In most cases admission of an infant to the neonatal unit is unexpected and is stressful for the parents.

If a problem is diagnosed antenatally, parents can be forewarned. For most admissions to the neonatal unit, however, there is little or no time to prepare the family. Parents are unfamiliar with the potentially complex problems their infant is facing and they are unsure of the future. Incomprehension and uncertainty are major sources of stress. In addition, maternal health is often compromised at this time.

A degree of separation exists between the mother and baby when the infant is admitted to the neonatal unit, and this may extend over many months. Although in some places a visit to the neonatal unit is a routine part of antenatal care, the neonatal unit is an alien environment to most parents. Units are often noisy, bright, and hot. They can be overcrowded and parts of every unit will be "high tech." Parents rarely know the neonatal unit staff before their baby is admitted, and the language and behaviours they encounter can contribute to an overwhelming feeling of isolation. The sickest preterm infants may be in hospital for many months, and visiting can be difficult, exhausting, and a financial drain for parents, especially as neonatal services become more centralised. All these factors put strain on the parents' relationship: breakdown is more common in couples during the months after preterm delivery. Some couples, however, feel the experience makes their relationship closer, at least initially.

Generally, stress and anxiety are higher in mothers than in fathers, and lessen as time goes by. In some parents stress is similar to that seen in adults diagnosed with post-traumatic stress disorder. High levels of stress may last beyond the first year of their infant's life, and the level and duration of stress may not be directly related to how preterm or how sick their baby is. In addition to high levels of stress and anxiety, these parents are more prone to clinical depression, which may be difficult to recognise.

Coping mechanisms

Responses and feelings reminiscent of a classic grief reaction can be identified: shock, denial, anger, guilt, acceptance, and adjustment. Several models explore how parents cope with having their baby in the neonatal unit. A great variety of mechanisms are seen, however, and a single model will

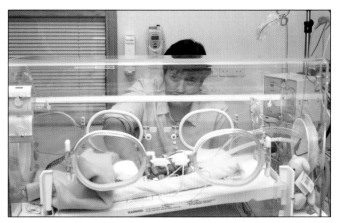

Seeing their baby receive intensive care can be terrifying for parents

Sources of stress experienced by parents

- Maternal ill health
- Separation from their baby
- Strange, "hostile" environment
- Unfamiliar staff
- Appearance and condition of the baby
- Complex medical problems to understand
- Sudden changes
- Uncertainty
- Lack of information
- Physical demands
- Financial hardship

The degree of stress and anxiety experienced by parents varies from individual to individual and with time

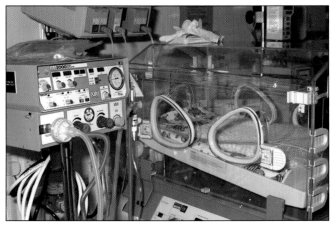

The environment of the neonatal intensive care unit, which can be hot, noisy and "high tech," is usually alien to parents

Cultural and religious variations may cause differences in the way experience of having a baby in the neonatal unit and the surrounding circumstances may be perceived and handled. Staff should be aware of this diversity so as not to view different responses by the parents as necessarily "abnormal" or uncaring

probably not fit all parents. Some of the coping strategies include trying to gain a deeper understanding of the problems, establishing a degree of control over the situation, seeking social support from other people, and escaping from or minimising the apparent severity of the situation. These mechanisms are used to varying degrees in individual parents, and there is a systematic difference seen between mothers and fathers. Mothers tend to look for support from others and to search for an explanation for what has happened, whereas fathers are more likely to try to minimise the situation, often by concentrating on supporting their partner.

Limiting parental stress

A better understanding of the sources of stress and how parents might try to cope allows appropriate care of the family. When designing neonatal units, great emphasis is placed on effective layout, lighting, and noise reduction. Facilities for families to stay close to their baby are usually provided, and parent rooms allow mothers and fathers to relax and meet other parents. Play areas for siblings can be incorporated into some units. This more "family-orientated" approach to care is helped by less restricted visiting policies in neonatal units. Most units will allow parents and siblings open access to their baby if they comply with local infection control measures. Having transitional care areas as an integral part of the neonatal unit or as a separate area (for example, as part of the postnatal ward) minimises the separation of mother and baby.

When time permits, members of the neonatal team will often meet with parents before the birth to discuss any likely admission. Parents may visit the unit before their baby is born to familiarise themselves with the environment and some of the staff. After delivery, it is good practice to discuss medical and nursing issues in detail with parents and to involve them in decision making from an early stage. Parents will often have immediate access to recordings, results, and clinical notes. They can also help care for their preterm baby. This care may extend beyond simple but important measures, such as "skin to skin" contact, to providing skilled care such as tube feeding, oral toileting, and intensive "developmental care" programmes.

Parents of other preterm babies can give personal support through "buddying" programmes or informally. Counselling through organisations, such as the Premature Baby Charity (BLISS) in the United Kingdom, or formal support can be helpful even for families whose babies are not critically ill. Written information about the neonatal unit and, where appropriate, describing specific conditions or procedures may be useful. Routine contact between the neonatal unit and social services may allow financial support to be provided for the parents.

Death and decision making

Babies, particularly extremely preterm infants, may die despite continuing intensive treatment and full medical support. In addition, a decision to limit active treatment may be made because of the inevitability of death or a prognosis that indicates a very poor quality of life. Death, however it comes about, is a desperate time for the families who are affected. Parents want to be involved in decision making at these times. They need full and frank information, given in a compassionate manner by experienced staff who know the family and their baby.

In most cases, the decision to stop or limit treatment is made with senior medical and nursing staff. Family, friends, and external bodies (such as religious leaders and support groups)

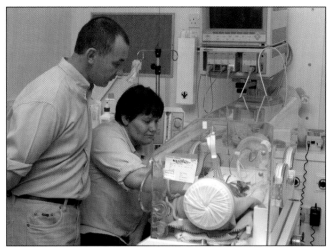
Fathers and mothers may respond to and deal with the stress of preterm birth differently

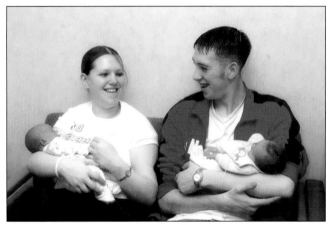
A place to relax as a family in the neonatal unit can help reduce stress and anxiety

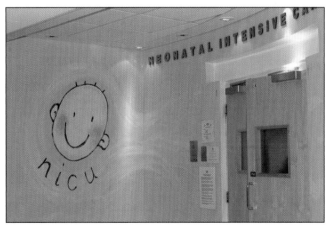
A welcoming environment is important in the neonatal intensive care unit

Effective bereavement support
- Compassionate, sensitive, caring environment where patients feel safe to grieve
- Support for siblings, grandparents, and other family members
- Opportunity to say goodbye to their baby
- Practical help—for example, with funeral arrangements
- Opportunity to ask questions
- Support for caregivers

do not often have a substantial role in the decision to withdraw treatment but they do contribute to family support afterwards.

Mothers and fathers may differ in the way they grieve and cope with their loss. Mementoes, formal contact with senior staff in the weeks after the death, and contact with a bereavement support worker or group may all help the process. Most families begin to move on in the first year after the death—not forgetting the child but adjusting to life without him or her.

Bereaved parents often need factual information that may help explain why their baby has died. Without autopsy, important information can be missed, and in most neonatal units, postmortem examination will always be considered and offered to the parents if appropriate. High profile cases of procedural inadequacies and anxieties about organ retention have contributed to a fall in the number of autopsies carried out. This drop is increased by a parent's natural reluctance to authorise further "suffering" for their infant and a lack of awareness of the questions that remain unanswered.

Discharge home

Discharge home, although an exciting time for families, can also be a time of extreme anxiety, and so a formal approach to "discharge planning" is often adopted. Mothers "room in" with their baby to promote bonding, establish feeding, and learn practical skills that might be needed. Support for the family in the community once the infant is discharged can also be arranged, including specialist neonatal nurses, primary care health staff (for example, health visitors, general practitioners), social workers, and national or local family support groups (for example, BLISS).

Although managing the immediate stress of discharge home is important, it needs to be recognised that although practical issues may become easier to manage as time passes, for some families considerable levels of stress and anxiety remain long after the discharge itself. Psychological support should be an integral part of neonatal follow up programmes.

Conclusion

The parents and families of babies who are admitted to the neonatal unit are exposed to a variety of stressors, and may face extremely difficult decisions in unique situations. Vulnerable families may benefit from specific environmental and personal support. By targeting this support appropriately, staff on neonatal units can provide a more complete package of care.

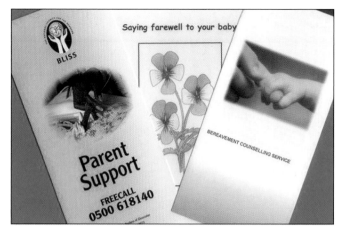

Leaflets are another source of support and information for parents and families

A formal approach to discharge planning has allowed infants who might otherwise have stayed in hospital for some time (for example, infants with chronic lung disease) to be discharged sooner to the more natural and stimulating home environment

Summary points

- Having a preterm baby is stressful
- Parents manage stress and anxiety in many ways that are not necessarily consistent across different families, religions, and cultures
- Men and women differ in how they cope with stress and bereavement
- Appropriate support for parents should be an integral part of neonatal care

Further reading

- Affleck G, Tennen H. The effect of newborn intensive care on parents' psychological well-being. *Child Health Care* 1991;20:6-14
- Harrison H. The principles for family-centered neonatal care. *Pediatrics* 1993;92:643-50
- Miles MS, Holditch-Davis D. Parenting the prematurely born child: pathways of influence. *Semin Perinatol* 1997;21:254-66
- Singer LT, Salvator A, Guo S, Collin M, Lilien L, Baley J. Maternal psychological distress and parenting stress after the birth of a very low-birth-weight infant. *JAMA* 1999;281:799-805
- McHaffie HE, Fowlie PW. *Life, death and decisions: doctors and nurses reflect on neonatal practice.* Hale: Hochland and Hochland, 1996
- McHaffie HE, Fowlie PW, Hume R, Laing I, Lloyd D, Lyon A. *Crucial decisions at the beginning of life: parents' experiences of treatment withdrawal from infants.* Oxford: Radcliffe Medical Press, 2001

11 Neurodevelopmental outcomes after preterm birth

Michael Colvin, William McGuire, Peter W Fowlie

The major clinical outcomes that are important to preterm infants and their families are survival and normal long term neurodevelopment. In developed countries over the past 30 years, better perinatal care has considerably improved these outcomes. This article covers the prevalence of neurodevelopmental problems and their types.

Prevalence

For most preterm infants of > 32 weeks' gestation, survival and longer term neurodevelopment are similar to those of infants born at term. Overall, outcomes are also good for infants born after shorter gestations. Most infants survive without substantial neurodevelopmental problems and most go on to attend mainstream schools, ultimately living independent lives.

A few preterm babies, however, do develop important and lasting neurodevelopmental problems. The period between 20 and 32 weeks after conception is one of rapid brain growth and development. Illness, undernutrition, and infection during this time may compromise neurodevelopment. The clinical consequences can include serious neuromotor problems (principally cerebral palsy), visual and hearing impairments, learning difficulties, and psychological, behavioural, and social problems.

Most substantial impairment occurs in the 0.2% of infants born before 28 weeks' gestation, or with birth weights of < 1000 g (extremely low birth weight). The survival rate for extremely preterm infants has improved over the past decade, but the overall prevalence of neurodisability after preterm birth has not fallen. In a recent North American follow up study of extremely low birthweight infants, one quarter of the children had neurological abnormalities when examined at 18 to 22 months post term.

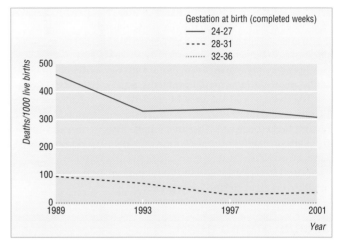

Neonatal death rate for preterm infants in Scotland since 1989 (deaths per 1000 live births by gestational age band). Adapted from Scottish perinatal and infant mortality and morbidity report, 2001

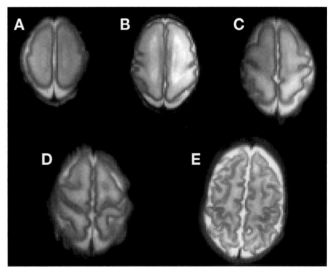

Brain growth and development of sulcation and gyration with increasing gestational age. Magnetic resonance images at the level of the central sulcus at: (A) 25 weeks; (B) 28 weeks; (C) 30 weeks; (D) 33 weeks; and (E) 39 weeks. With permission from Counsell SJ et al. *Arch Dis Child* 2003;88:269-74

Prevalence of neuromotor and sensory findings at 18 months in extremely low birthweight infants*

Abnormal neurological examination—25%
- Cerebral palsy—17%
- Seizure disorder—5%
- Hydrocephalus with shunt—4%

Any vision impairment—9%
- Unilateral blindness—1%
- Bilateral blindness—2%

Hearing impairment—11%
- Wears hearing aids—3%

*Adapted from Vohr BR et al. *Paediatrics* 2000;105:1216-26

In the United Kingdom, the EPICure Study Group has evaluated outcomes for surviving infants born before 26 weeks' gestation. At a median age of 30 months (corrected for gestational age), about half the children had disability and about half of these children had severe disability. Severe disability is defined as impairments that will probably put the child in need of assistance to perform daily activities. The prevalence of disability remained high when the children were reassessed at 6 years, with less than half of them having no evidence of impairment.

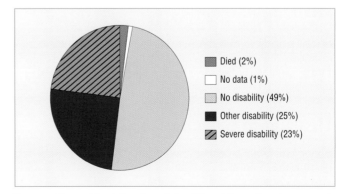

Died (2%)
No data (1%)
No disability (49%)
Other disability (25%)
Severe disability (23%)

Outcomes for surviving infants born before 26 weeks' gestation when assessed at 30 months. Adapted from Wood NS et al. *N Engl J Med* 2000;343:378-84

Cerebral palsy

Most children with cerebral palsy were not born preterm. However, preterm infants, particularly those born after very short gestations, are at increased risk of cerebral palsy. Additional specific perinatal risk factors for cerebral palsy in preterm infants include feto-maternal infection, neonatal sepsis, and other severe illness in the newborn period.

Brain damage related to periventricular haemorrhage, particularly periventricular cystic leucomalacia and posthaemorrhagic hydrocephalus are strong predictors of future neurodevelopmental problems, especially cerebral palsy.

The most common forms of cerebral palsy in children who have been born preterm are spastic hemiplegia (unilateral) or quadriplegia (bilateral). The functional consequences can vary from abnormalities of muscle tone or power that do not cause serious problems, to severe impairments that result in considerable lifelong disability and handicap, such as being unable to walk or to feed independently.

Visual impairment

Most visual impairment in very preterm infants is secondary to retinopathy of prematurity, although some cases are caused by cortical damage. Retinopathy of prematurity affects infants born at < 32 weeks' gestation. The incidence and severity is inversely related to gestational age. The risk seems to be directly related to the concentration and the duration of oxygen treatment to which the very preterm infant is exposed. Relative hyperoxia (compared with the hypoxic intrauterine environment) disturbs normal retinal vascular development in preterm infants. Careful use of supplemental oxygen treatment, with monitoring of the blood oxygen saturation and partial pressure, may prevent severe retinopathy in many infants. The ideal target range of saturation or partial pressure of oxygen in very preterm infants is unclear.

Most infants born at < 28 weeks' gestation will develop some form of retinopathy. In most cases this is mild and regresses spontaneously. Some infants, however, develop progressive retinopathy with abnormal vessel growth, retinal haemorrhage, scarring, and detachment. As outcome is improved with early treatment, infants born at < 32 weeks' gestation or with birth weights of < 1500 g should be screened for early signs of the disease by an ophthalmologist. Screening should continue at least fortnightly until vascularisation has progressed to the outer retina, with progressive retinopathy being treated with either cryotherapy or laser photocoagulation.

Although the incidence and severity of retinopathy of prematurity has fallen in developed countries over the past 20 years, it remains one of the commonest causes of childhood blindness, visual field defects, and refractive errors. Despite screening and treatment, about 2% of extremely low birthweight infants are blind as a result of retinopathy of prematurity. The incidence is increasing in some countries, especially "middle income" countries in Latin America, Eastern Europe, and South East Asia that have introduced neonatal intensive care services for preterm infants.

Hearing impairment

About 3% of infants born at < 28 weeks' gestation require hearing aids, though more infants have milder hearing impairment or high frequency hearing loss. The aetiology of sensorineural hearing loss is probably multifactorial, with a variety of interacting factors that are related to illness severity

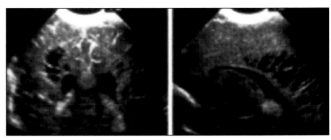

Cranial ultrasonography: (left) coronal and (right) parasagittal views on day 24 in an infant born at 28 weeks' gestation, showing extensive periventricular cysts. With permission from Pierrat V et al. *Arch Dis Child* 2001;84:151-6

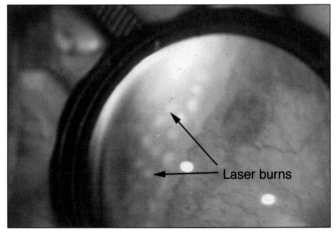

Magnified view of laser treatment of retinopathy of prematurity

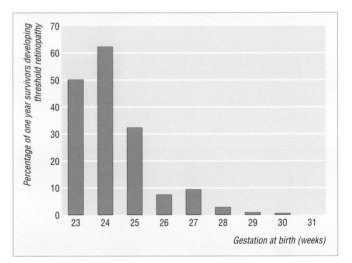

Incidence of severe retinopathy and its relation to gestation at birth. Adapted from Pennefather PM et al. *Eye* 1995;9:26-30

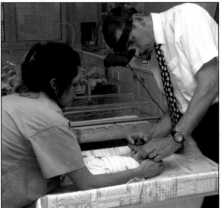

Screening for retinopathy of prematurity

contributing. Hearing impairment is associated with delayed language development, although very preterm infants with normal hearing may also develop speech and language problems. Early use of hearing aids plus support from audiology services can improve language development in infants with sensorineural hearing loss.

Learning difficulties

At school age, up to 50% of infants born before 28 weeks' gestation need some form of additional educational support. A recent systematic review found that the IQ of extremely low birthweight children is on average 10 points lower than in children who were born at term. Learning difficulties are often associated with problems such as visual or hearing impairment, but children can have isolated cognitive problems. Very preterm children of normal intelligence may have specific learning difficulties, commonly with mathematics or reading. Confounding social factors (for example, mother's educational status) may have a greater influence on educational outcome than extremely preterm birth.

Social development, behaviour, and psychological problems

Early social development—for example, responsive smiling and recognising family members—may be delayed in preterm infants. Interactive and imaginative play may also be delayed. Investigators from several countries have noted a higher incidence of behavioural problems in extremely low birthweight children of school age, with attention, social, and thought processing problems the most commonly detected. As behavioural problems can adversely affect school performance and development of social relations, these are important long term effects of preterm birth.

Quality of life

In the last decade, data from cohort studies have indicated that quality of life related to health (measured using validated tools) is considerably lower in surviving extremely low birthweight children than in children born at term. Evidence exists, however, that most children do not perceive their quality of life as being substantially different from that of their peers born at term.

Neurodevelopmental follow up

Regular follow up assessments of children at risk of neurodevelopmental impairment may allow the early detection of problems and the provision of medical, social, and educational support if required. Many signs of neurodevelopmental impairment are evident only after infancy, and follow up should continue until the child is at least 18-24 months old, corrected for gestation. Standardised, validated assessment tools to monitor developmental progress are available. Ideally, these follow up data should be included in the annual audit of activity and outcomes of neonatal units. Even in well resourced centres, it is often difficult to undertake comprehensive follow up programmes.

Data on the longer term neurodevelopmental outcomes are important for informing the antenatal counselling of mothers who may deliver preterm, especially at the limits of viability (<26 weeks' gestation). National, population-based data are most valid. The number of extremely preterm infants cared for

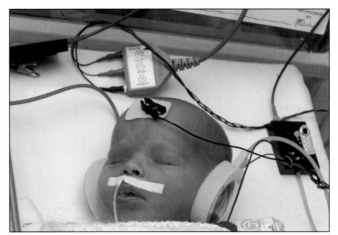

Preterm infants at risk of hearing loss should be screened, usually with brainstem auditory evoked responses, before discharge from the neonatal unit

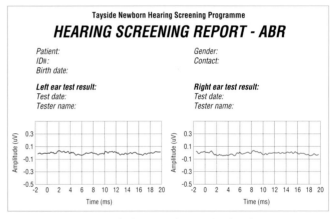

Screening audiogram that indicates possible hearing impairment and referral for further assessment

Children, their parents, other parents and, importantly, healthcare workers may all view similar health states differently

---

Benefits of neurodevelopmental follow up

- Early detection of problems in individual children
- Prognostic information for families can be provided
- Allows audit of outcomes for neonatal units and health services

---

in each unit is small, and estimates of the incidence of outcomes are often imprecise. At present, such population-based data are mainly available through research studies, such as the EPICure study. In some countries routine collection and synthesis of such data is being attempted—for example, using nationally agreed minimum datasets reporting standardised assessments.

Conclusion

Most preterm infants have good neurodevelopmental outcomes and cannot readily be distinguished from term infants. As survival rates for extremely preterm infants have improved, however, the overall number of preterm infants with disability and handicap has not fallen as might have been expected. These impairments may have an adverse effect on family life as well as having an important impact on social, education, and health service resources. The longer term neurodevelopmental outcomes must be considered when reviewing the impact of neonatal intensive care for preterm infants.

Further reading

- Marlow N, Wolke D, Bracewell MA, Samara M. Neurologic and Developmental disability at 6 years of age after extremely pre-term birth. The EPICure Study Group. *N Engl J Med* 2005;352:9-19
- Wood NS, Marlow N, Costeloe K, Gibson AT, Wilkinson AR. Neurologic and developmental disability after extremely preterm birth. EPICure Study Group. *N Engl J Med.* 2000;343:378-84
- Costeloe K, Henness E, Gibson AT, Marlow N, Wilkinson AR. The EPICure study: outcomes to discharge from hospital for infants born at the threshold of viability. *Pediatrics* 2000;106:659-71
- Bhutta AT, Cleves MA, Casey PH, Cradock MM, Anand KJ. Cognitive and behavioural outcomes of school-aged children who were born preterm: a meta-analysis. *JAMA* 2002;288:728-37
- Donohue PK. Health-related quality of life of preterm children and their caregivers. *Ment Retard Dev Disabil Res Rev* 2002;8:293-7
- Wheatley CM, Dickinson JL, Mackey DA, Craig JE, Surrell MM. Retinopathy of prematurity: recent advances in our understanding. *Arch Dis Child* 2002; 87:78-82
- Saigal S. Follow-up of very low birthweight babies to adolescence. *Semin Neonatol* 2000;5:107-18

The magnified view of laser treatment of retinopathy of prematurity is with permission from Nick George, Ninewells Hospital, Dundee. The chart showing neonatal death rate for preterm infants in Scotland since 1989 is adapted from the Scottish perinatal and infant mortality and morbidity report 2001, which can be found on the website www.isdscotland.org

12   Evidence based care

Peter Brocklehurst, William McGuire

The ethos of basing practice on the best available evidence is well established in perinatal medicine. The introduction to clinical practice of major interventions, such as antenatal corticosteroids and exogenous surfactant, was informed by evidence from seminal randomised controlled trials and systematic reviews.

Equally important has been the development and evaluation of interventions that have been shown not to have major benefits for preterm infants. For example, strong evidence from preclinical research studies indicated that antenatal thyrotropin releasing hormone might act synergistically with corticosteroids to reduce the risk of respiratory distress syndrome in preterm infants. Despite the biological plausibility of this treatment and evidence of effect in animal models, randomised controlled trials (involving over 4500 women) did not show any improvement in outcomes, including mortality, for preterm infants. Also, antenatal thyrotropin releasing hormone was shown to be associated with adverse effects for mothers and infants, including a higher risk of infants needing mechanical ventilation. On the basis of this evidence, antenatal thyrotropin releasing hormone does not have a role in the management of threatened preterm birth.

Evidence

Obtaining the best evidence to guide clinical practice is not always easy. In particular, undertaking clinical trials to evaluate interventions for preterm infants is difficult. Although about 3000 randomised controlled trials have been reported in the field of neonatology, many interventions have not yet been subjected to unbiased evaluation. This could be because the trials have not been attempted, or have been flawed methodologically, or have been too small to detect clinically important effects. Large perinatal trials have problems with recruitment. This could be related to the issues surrounding the public perception of perinatal trials and the need for (and difficulty in obtaining) informed consent from parents. Even when perinatal trials have been undertaken successfully, in some studies follow up has been too short and has assessed short term or surrogate outcomes for preterm infants.

Difficulties in undertaking randomised controlled trials

- Limited infrastructure to support studies
- Large trials needed to detect modest effect sizes—trials need to be multicentre or multinational, or both
- Limited funding—perinatal health not viewed as a funding priority
- Limited potential for industrial partnership
- Trial recruitment undertaken by busy clinicians or carers
- Validity of informed consent obtained at stressful times
- Public perception of perinatal research
- Need for long term follow up

The need for large trials

The introduction of antenatal steroids and exogenous surfactants is associated with about a 40% reduction in the risk of mortality. Future interventions for preterm infants will probably not have the same major beneficial effects as each of these interventions. Future trials must be designed to detect much more modest (but

---

> **Evidence based practice—the integration of individual clinical expertise with the best available clinical evidence from systematic research**   **David Sackett**

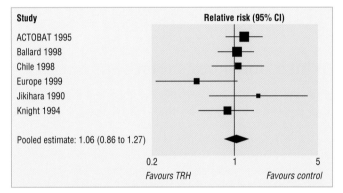

Effect of prenatal thyrotropin releasing hormone (TRH) for preterm birth on mortality before hospital discharge. Data from Crowther CA et al. *Cochrane Database Syst Rev.* 2003;(4): CD000019

Levels of evidence for effects of treatments—limiting bias

- Systematic review of all relevant randomised controlled trials
- Large multicentre randomised controlled trials
- Controlled trials without randomisation
- Cohort studies
- Case controlled studies
- Multiple time series
- Before and after studies
- Opinions based on clinical experience or expert committee

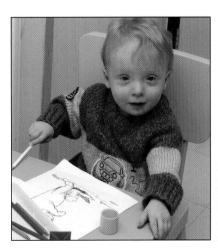

Evidence based care should be informed by the best quality evidence for the effect of interventions on clinically important longer term outcomes

clinically important) effects. These trials will have to recruit many mothers and infants, and be multicentre, and often multinational. Despite problems with infrastructure, support, and public perception, recent randomised controlled trials have provided answers to important questions for preterm infants, their families, and carers.

In some places—for example, in North America and Australasia—perinatal networks for undertaking multicentre trials are well established. In the United Kingdom and other countries, an administrative infrastructure for protocol development, data management, and follow up in perinatal trials needs do be formalised. Collaborative networks of perinatal units undertaking large trials will allow parent groups and researchers to prioritise their most important questions. These collaborations also ensure that competing trials do not occur simultaneously. If perinatal care is to continue to improve outcomes, all potential new interventions for preterm infants must be assessed in the most efficient way.

Which outcomes should we measure?

Trials must evaluate outcomes that are important to infants and their families as well as to carers and health services. To date, the major question for many interventions has been: "Does this treatment improve the chances of survival?" As advances in care of preterm infants have reduced mortality, however, the effect of interventions on morbidity in surviving infants must be considered. This is particularly important in perinatal practice as there is a potential for interventions to improve short term outcomes but also to increase the likelihood of adverse longer term outcomes in surviving infants. For example, giving preterm infants systemic corticosteroids in the first few days of postnatal life improves short term respiratory outcomes, such as allowing earlier weaning from the ventilator or reducing oxygen dependency. Trials that undertook longer term follow up, however, showed that infants who received corticosteroids had a higher rate of adverse neurological effects, including cerebral palsy.

The importance of assessing outcomes that are relevant to infants and families rather than surrogate outcomes is further illustrated by the trials of tocolytic drugs used to suppress uterine contractions and delay preterm delivery. Trials assessing these treatments have usually measured gestation at delivery as a primary outcome. Meta-analysis of these trials showed an unequivocal effect of tocolytic drugs delaying delivery. Although there is a strong relation between length of gestation and the risk of neonatal mortality and morbidity, it does not necessarily follow that delaying delivery improves important outcomes for infants. In fact, meta-analyses of trials of tocolysis have not showed any effect on perinatal mortality or morbidity, but they have shown a higher risk of maternal adverse effects. Further large randomised controlled trials with long term follow up are needed to assess if tocolysis is a benign intervention for mothers and preterm infants.

Evaluating the longer term neurodevelopmental outcomes of perinatal treatments is difficult and expensive. Abnormal motor function or severe neurosensory disability can be assessed in the second year after birth, but milder sensory problems, or behavioural problems, are more reliably assessed in older preschool children. Educational and cognitive deficits are not apparent until children are of school age. Follow up of trial cohorts must be as complete as possible as children who are difficult to follow up have a higher risk of impairment than those who are easily found.

Recent examples of large perinatal trials

Trial	Main question	Participants
CRYO-ROP (follow up)	Do the benefits of cryotherapy for threshold retinopathy of prematurity persist into later childhood?	247 children evaluated at aged 10 years (97% follow up)
TIPPS	Does indomethacin prophylaxis affect long term neurological outcomes for extremely low birthweight infants?	1202 extremely low birthweight infants from 32 centres in five countries
ORACLE	Do maternal antibiotics improve perinatal outcomes in spontaneous preterm labour, or preterm, prelabour rupture of fetal membranes?	4826 women with preterm, prelabour rupture of fetal membranes; 6295 women in spontaneous preterm labour
BOOST	Does targeting a higher oxygen saturation range in preterm infants dependent on supplemental oxygen improve growth and development?	358 infants born at less than 30 weeks of gestation (dependent on supplemental oxygen at 32 weeks of postmenstrual age)
INIS	Does polyclonal immunoglobulin improve long term outcomes for neonates with sepsis?	Ongoing: planned to recruit 5000 infants
CAP	Does management of apnoea of prematurity without methylxanthines affect survival without neurodisability in very preterm infants?	Ongoing: aiming to enrol > 1000 infants weighing 500-1250 g at birth

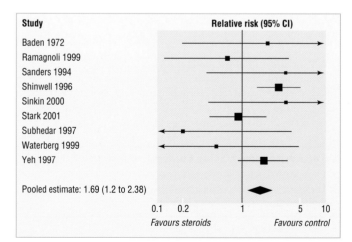

Effect of corticosteroids given in the first few days after birth in preterm infants on incidence of cerebral palsy in survivors. Adapted from Halliday HL et al. *Cochrane Database Syst Rev.* 2004(1): CD001146

The costs of tracking and assessing large groups of children for long periods need to be planned for in the development of trials

Informed consent

Informed consent is fundamental to giving legal and ethical protection to parents and preterm infants participating in research studies. Problems arise in gaining informed consent for interventions at or around the time of birth or during emergency treatment of an infant with a life threatening condition. In such circumstances it may be difficult to have a discussion in which the parents have time to consider their options and provide fully informed consent.

Qualitative research has indicated that parents value their part in the informed consent process. However, some evidence exists that current practice in obtaining valid consent for participation in perinatal trials is flawed, especially in circumstances when parents are approached at a stressful time, such as during an emergency situation. In several large perinatal trials parents have been informed antenatally about the possible need for emergency intervention around the time of birth. This approach, which allows parents to withdraw presumed consent at any stage thereafter, may help to increase recruitment rates without compromising parental understanding of the nature and purpose of the research. The elements of the consent process valued by parents and carers need to be identified.

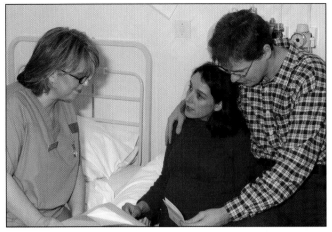

Recruitment of pregnant women into clinical trials is complicated because an intervention to which mother and child are exposed may cause harm as well as good

Getting evidence into practice

Bridging gaps between evidence and practice is central to ensuring that beneficial interventions are used appropriately, and harmful interventions are avoided. Busy clinicians, however, may not always be aware of all evidence based practice guidelines. Randomised controlled trials have indicated that strategies such as introducing guidelines via an opinion leader, organising group discussions and training workshops, and undertaking audit and performance feedback can promote the use of the best available evidence.

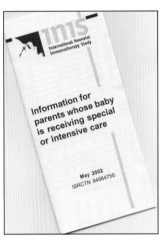

Written information and talking to parents can help improve their understanding of the research process

Conclusion

Well conducted randomised controlled trials can provide the least biased assessment of interventions to improve outcomes for preterm infants. Increasingly, these trials will be large, multicentre, international, use a simple and pragmatic protocol, and incorporate good follow up and assessment of long term outcomes. To achieve good quality research, it is essential to continue to engage with parents and patients. Care of the preterm infants is a rapidly changing field and there are frequent shifts in the weight of accumulating evidence. Systematic reviews of the results of randomised trials must be updated continuously so that the evidence base from which the clinical guidelines are developed remains valid.

Further reading

- Leviton LC, Goldenberg RL, Baker CS, Swartz RM, Freda MC, Fish LJ, et al. Methods to encourage the use of antenatal corticosteroid therapy for fetal maturation: a randomized controlled trial. *JAMA* 1999;281:46-52
- Horbar JD, Carpenter JH, Buzas J, Soll RF, Suresh G, Bracken MB, et al. Collaborative quality improvement to promote evidence based surfactant for preterm infants: a cluster randomised trial. *BMJ* 2004;329:1004
- Field D. Evidence in perinatal medicine: enough of trial and error? *Arch Dis Child Fetal Neonatal Ed* 1999;81:F161
- Manning DJ. Presumed consent in emergency neonatal research. *J Med Ethics* 2000;26:249-53
- Mason SA, Allmark PJ. Obtaining informed consent to neonatal randomised controlled trials: interviews with parents and clinicians in the Euricon study. *Lancet* 2000;356:2045-51
- Tin W, Fritz S, Wariyar U, Hey E. Outcome of very preterm birth: children reviewed with ease at 2 years differ from those followed up with difficulty. *Arch Dis Child Fetal Neonatal Ed* 1998;79:F83-87

Index

Notes: As preterm birth is the subject of this book, all index entries refer to preterm birth unless otherwise indicated. Page references in *italics* refer to figures, tables or boxed material.

Index